MORE PRAISE FOR BOOKS
BY CHARLES R. MORRIS

The Surgeons

"An ambitious account of the complicated interplay among health care economics, policy and those individuals whose professional lives drive the medical system. Morris fully immerses himself, and the reader, in the complexities of health care. . . . In the final chapters of the book, Morris steps back, superimposing his clinical observations upon the larger issues of health care policy and economics. . . . His chapter on the controversies surrounding aprotinin, an antibleeding agent often used in cardiac surgery, is particularly impressive. . . . What ultimately brings clarity to this book—and hope for health care reform—are the stories Morris delivers along the way."

—Pauline W. Chen, *New York Times Book Review*

"The stories are insightful and filled with verve. There is the electrifying late-night 'harvest run' to secure a donor heart, the day-to-day frenzy of a heart surgeon in training, and the poignant death of a child from a failed heart transplant. ('The entire kit of marvels mustered by cardiologists and surgeons in three states had not been up to the task of saving her.')"   —*Wall Street Journal*

"By embedding himself in a frontline unit, Charles Morris has captured the real-life stories of cardiac surgeons and their patients. Told with the drama and pace of television fiction, this book offers an unprecedented look at the surgeons who hold our hearts in their hands."   —Paul Offit, author of *Vaccinated: One Man's Quest to Defeat the World's Deadliest Diseases*

"Poignant and extraordinary."   —*Herald* (Glasgow)

"Charles Morris has written an astute book of enormous importance: an inside look at cardiac surgery as done in a great university medical center, written by an outsider so keenly observant, of such understanding and perceptiveness, that he has earned the frank trust and cooperation of the very surgeons whose work he scrutinizes with such perceptive eyes and ears. This is a book worthy to take its place alongside the works of such physicians as Jerome Groopman and Atul Gawande, and such social scientists as Renee Fox and Charles Bosk."

—Sherwin Nuland, author of *The Art of Aging: A Doctor's Prescription for Well-Being*

"[Morris] writes like the best professor you ever had—no dumbing down, presenting complex material in an engaging manner with just the right story at just the right time. If the term 'public intellectual' did not exist, it would have to be invented for Morris. . . . *The Surgeons* takes on all the key issues—the increasing costs of medical care, the differences between American medical care and that of other Western nations, suggestions for improving American medical care, the roles of the pharmaceutical industry and the F.D.A., the conflicts over the best way to test and measure drugs and medicines and hospitals. . . . In unison with earlier public intellectuals now regarded as sages—Galen, Aristotle, Maimonides—Morris reminds us that good medicine can flourish only in a good society."

—James R. Kelly, *America*

"From detailing the workings of the heart's chambers and valves to the bald economics of cardiac surgery . . . Morris masterfully breaks down complex jargon, procedures and policies for a lay audience."

—*Publishers Weekly*

The Trillion Dollar Meltdown:
Easy Money, High Rollers, and the Great Credit Crash
A *New York Times* Bestseller

"How we got into the mess we're in, explained briefly and brilliantly."   —*New York Times Book Review*, Editors' Choice

"An absolutely excellent narrative of the horror that we have in the credit markets right now."   —Paul Steiger

"The first big book on the credit crunch. . . . This provocative book is . . . a well-aimed opening shot in a debate that will only grow louder in coming months."   —*Economist*

The Tycoons: How Andrew Carnegie,
John D. Rockefeller, Jay Gould, and J. P. Morgan
Invented the American Supereconomy

"Engaging and credible."   —*Washington Post*

"Makes the reader feel like a time traveler plopped down among men both vicious and visionary. . . . Looks back with clarity at the Big Bang of the American boom."   —*Christian Science Monitor*

The Cost of Good Intentions:
New York City and the Liberal Experiment, 1960–1975

"This is the most complete, lucid, and thoughtful chronicle yet written about the city's fiscal crisis. . . . But by tracing what city officials thought was happening, as well as what was really happening, Mr. Morris has produced something more, a meticulous case study of 'good intentions' gone awry."   —Steve Weisman, *New York Times Book Review*

THE
SURGEONS

*Life and Death in
a Top Heart Center*

CHARLES R. MORRIS

W. W. NORTON & COMPANY

NEW YORK

The illustrations on pages 270–271 are from *Mayo Clinic Heart Book*,
Second Edition, by Bernard J. Gersh. Copyright © 1993, 2000 by Mayo
Foundation for Medical Education and Research.
Reprinted by permission of HarperCollins Publishers.

For information about permission to reproduce selections from this book,
write to Permissions, W. W. Norton & Company, Inc.,
500 Fifth Avenue, New York, NY 10110

For information about special discounts for bulk purchases, please contact
W. W. Norton Special Sales at specialsales@wwnorton.com or 800-233-4830

Manufacturing by RR Donnelley, Bloomsburg
Book design by Lovedog Studio
Production manager: Anna Oler

Library of Congress Cataloging-in-Publication Data

Morris, Charles R.
The surgeons : life and death in a top heart center / Charles R. Morris.—1st ed.
p. ; cm.
Includes bibliographical references and index.
ISBN 978-0-393-06562-6 (hardcover)
1. Columbia University Medical Center. 2. Heart—Surgery—New York
(State)—New York—History. 3. Heart surgeons—New York
(State)—New York—Biography. I. Title.
[DNLM: 1. Columbia University Medical Center. 2. Academic Medical
Centers—history—New York City—Personal Narratives. 3. Thoracic
Surgery—history—New York City—Personal Narratives. 4. Cardiac Surgical
Procedures—New York City—Personal Narratives. 5. Health Policy—
trends—New York City—Personal Narratives. WG 28 M875s 2007]
RD598.M579 2007
617.092—dc22
[B]

2007024227

ISBN 978-0-393-33423-4 pbk.

W. W. Norton & Company, Inc., 500 Fifth Avenue, New York, N.Y. 10110
www.wwnorton.com

W. W. Norton & Company Ltd., Castle House, 75/76 Wells Street, W1T 3QT

1 2 3 4 5 6 7 8 9 0

For Kathleen, Jenn, and Hiro

CONTENTS

PREFACE

I BECAME INTERESTED IN WRITING ABOUT HEARTS after running across a snippet of data showing that the United States now spends more on treating and repairing hearts than on new passenger cars—a straw in the wind, it seemed, that warranted further exploration.

I'd been intermittently involved in health care businesses and have occasionally written on health care policy issues, but I had no preconceived idea for a book, except that I wanted to learn as much as I could about the "heart industry."

In the course of talking to people in the field, a lawyer friend, Joe Bartlett, who has been deeply involved in medical issues, offered to introduce me to Craig Smith, the chief of the heart and lung surgery division at Columbia-Presbyterian hospital in New York City. It is a premier cardiac surgery center, and the country's largest heart transplant center by a substantial margin.

After several discussions with Smith, he agreed that I

could "embed" within the division an extended period in order to get a ground-level view of its operation. I wanted to learn how doctors think about their profession and their business, the pressures they work under, how they make decisions, how they choose their colleagues, how they get paid. I was also curious about the play of outside forces—regulators, pharmaceutical and equipment companies, accrediting agencies, patients—on what the doctors do and how they do it. But I decided to drop any preconceptions for a book, immerse myself in the division, and let the book come to me.

Smith stipulated that there would necessarily be meetings I would be barred from attending, and topics that might be off-limits, which seemed reasonable enough. As a practical matter, once I had been with the division for several weeks, I became part of the wallpaper and could attend virtually any meeting at all and ask about anything, subject only to legal restrictions on patient privacy. I observed all or part of about two dozen operations and met a fairly large cross-section of patients. (I was always introduced to patients as a writer, but no one ever objected to my presence. That surprised me at first, but, on reflection, don't we all like to talk about our illnesses?) Smith himself proved an ideal interlocutor—available, open, straightforward, nondefensive, and self-critical.

There were many surprises. I had never understood how many details of an operation are decided only after the chest is open and the surgeon can see and touch the diseases he will be working on. Despite all the scientific understanding of the heart, the critical decisions always come down to what will work with *this* patient, *this* set of coronary arteries, *this* misshapen mitral valve. The image that kept springing to mind was that of the Renaissance violin maker—the combination of lore, empirical understanding, and the insight of genius that no machine or computer program has ever replicated.

Nor had I appreciated the speed with which technology is moving, or how fast the field is changing. I had never imagined that a heart center could routinely transplant two hearts a week, or how astonishingly high transplant survival rates are—or how close we are getting to the ideal of workable, relatively inexpensive artificial hearts. And I have a much better idea of why health care spending is growing so fast and why it will almost certainly continue to do so.

Everything I learned at Columbia-Presbyterian, however, came from watching stories unfold—a difficult operation, a resident's progress, a wrenching life-or-death decision. This book is a compilation of those stories.

ACKNOWLEDGMENTS

MY THANKS FIRST OF ALL TO CRAIG SMITH FOR giving me the run of the heart and lung surgery division, for never ducking a question, and for always giving a straight answer, no matter how it played. And to Marty Leon for giving me similar privileges for a shorter comparative tour in interventional cardiology. Then to Diane Amato, the heart and lung surgery division administrator, who always made sure that I was getting where I wanted to go, talking to whom I wanted to talk to, and finding the data I was looking for. And to the surgeons, anesthesiologists, cardiologists, fellows, and others—I won't list them here because they're all in the book—for allowing me to look over their shoulders as they worked and for tolerating my elementary-school questions about what they were doing and why. And finally to the administrative and managerial staff, especially Larry Bielis, Jennifer Quill, and Caroline Mahoney for countless daily facilitations of the project.

This is not an "authorized" book or a public-relations piece. Smith made it clear that I could write about what I saw, good or bad—and I do. No one at Columbia-Presbyterian read it in draft form, or even asked if they could. So I write not just about successful operations, but also about mistakes made and procedures gone sour. But to be equally honest, I make no effort to conceal the great admiration I developed for the skill, the dedication, the stamina, and the calmness with which these doctors, day after day, execute high-wire operations where, as one of them put it, sudden death is lurking "under every rock you turn over."

A number of friends read all or portions of the manuscript. Special thanks to Drs. Sherwin Nuland, Sam Kopel, and Jim Vogel for picking out multiple mistakes of comprehension or terminology; to Sherry Glied, especially for statistical insights; and to Mike Bessie, Chris Reid, Claude Singer, Andrew Kerr, Dick Leone, Leif Haass, and my wife, Beverly, for intelligent and patient readings.

It's a pleasure to be working again with Norton and Ed Barber—after more than a quarter century—and I appreciated Tom Mayer's careful and unobtrusive editing. And my thanks as always to my agent Tim Seldes at Russell & Volkening.

A note on usage: I prefer alternating indefinite singular pronouns to the clumsy "he or she" construction. In the case of the heart surgeons, however, I always use the "he" because they were in fact all male. It's good to report that Mona Flores began her training this past fall. She is the third female cardiothoracic resident—the first was almost thirty years ago—in Columbia-Presbyterian's history.

THE SURGEONS

Chapter 1

FIXING
MR. GOLDFARB

ROY GOLDFARB IS A RETIRED PHARMACY EXECUTIVE from Boca Raton, in his early seventies, a large, good-humored man with a lovely smile; he is also very sick. It is early February 2006, about seven-thirty in the morning, and I'm watching him being wheeled into a cardiac operating room at the New York–Presbyterian Hospital/Columbia University Medical Center in New York City, or "Columbia-Presbyterian," as the staff call it.

Operating rooms, "ORs," are alien places—all shining surfaces and blinking monitors in bright, dead light. Like most surgery patients, Goldfarb has been tranquilized for his trip to the OR, and with good reason: lying amid the liana forest of glistening tubes and wires, surrounded by masked figures, staring up at the intense surgical lamps, is akin to the nightmare fantasies of a UFO abductee. Goldfarb has also been warned by his surgeon, Craig Smith, that while this operation is viewed as a "safe" one, the chances of a "major adverse event"—death, a stroke, kidney failure—are about 4 to 5 percent. And since Goldfarb has had heart surgery before, he's had firsthand experience of the injuries that are about to be inflicted upon him. He knows that he will wake up hours later in major pain, that it will be some days before he will be able to get around by himself, that he will feel weak and exhausted for a month or more, and that some after-effects, like memory problems, could persist for a year. But he also knows that he has a diseased heart valve that has imposed an unsustainable burden on his heart, and that if he doesn't get it fixed, he'll die.

Like many heart patients, Goldfarb suffers from a variety of "comorbidities"—his speech is slightly slurred by Parkinson's, he has diabetes, and he takes at least a dozen prescription medications. But the reason his Florida cardiologist recommended that he fly to Columbia-Presbyterian for his operation is that he is a "reop." He had bypass surgery a dozen years before, and his chest images show large white smears of sticky postoperative scar tissue that pose special challenges for a surgeon.

Columbia-Presbyterian—along with the Cleveland Clinic, the Texas Heart Institute, and perhaps a dozen others—ranks among the elite cardiac surgery centers that regularly receive difficult cases from other heart centers. Heart surgery volumes have been trending down in the United States, but Columbia-Presbyterian's volumes rose strongly in 2005 to nearly 2,000 cases, about an 18 percent increase. It has special capabilities in pediatric surgery and performs more heart transplants than any other center in the United States. Smith has been chief of the cardiothoracic division for the past ten years, and has been on the

Columbia faculty for more than twenty. A former college football and lacrosse player, he is a lean and athletic-looking fifty-seven. Although he is reserved almost to the point of shyness, Smith is a fine public speaker and found himself much in the public eye in 2004, including a stint on *Larry King Live*, after he performed a quadruple bypass operation on former President Bill Clinton. Smith's name shows up consistently on "best doctor'" lists, and he was recently chosen "practitioner of the year" by Columbia's physician association. In early 2007, he received a special honor from the American Heart Association for his "contributions to cardiovascular medicine and science." Clinton himself made an unannounced appearance to present the award. He said presenting it made him the happiest person in the room "because I'm still alive."

Surgical repair of human hearts first became practical in the early post–World War II era, and the techniques spread rapidly in the 1960s. Heart surgery set the pattern for the spectacular high-tech American style of attacking disease—spectacular in execution and expense, but often in results as well. The heart was the ideal early target. Its detailed physiology is still being unraveled, but in principle it is the simplest of organs: a four-chamber pump that operates much like any other pump. It is also very hard to break, because its electrical engine is distributed through every cell of the myocardium, the thick wall of muscle that surrounds the heart's chambers. ("Myocardium" is Latinized Greek for "heart muscle," a remnant of the old expectation that doctors speak Latin.) Myocardial cells are uniquely designed to beat, and only to beat, for as long as they live; drop them into a petri dish, and they beat all by themselves—it's just what they do. The heart can therefore withstand the grossest of insults—cut into a heart, stick tubes into it, twist it into a ball—and for the most part it keeps on beating.

The heart's pumping sequence is straightforward. The right side of the heart collects blood from the venous system and pumps it into the lungs to be reoxygenated. The left side collects blood from the lungs and pumps it through the body. Each side has two chambers—an atrium where blood is collected, and a ventricle that does the pumping work. The largest and most muscled chamber is the left ventricle, for it must deliver the powerful contractile thrust that drives the blood, up to six gallons a minute, through thousands of miles of vessels before it returns to the right atrium for recharging. While healthy circulation requires that all four chambers work well, failures in the left ventricle are usually the most immediately life-threatening, and the most frequent targets of surgical interventions.*

The valve that brought Goldfarb to the OR is his aortic valve. It sits at the crucial junction where blood flows from the left ventricle into the aorta, the sluiceway into the body's arterial system. The aorta is an enormous blood vessel that rises several inches straight up out of the heart and then arches sharply downward. The valve is a simple ring with three overlapping flaps that are locked in the closed position until they are blasted open by the surge of blood from the ventricle. The ejected blood fires through the valve straight up into the aorta, hits the arch, and bounces

*See Appendix I for schematics of the heart.

back on the valve flaps, slamming them shut—an elegantly simple and efficient design. Goldfarb's valve, however, is encrusted with thick deposits of calcium that prevent it from fully opening at the outward surge or fully closing on the bounce-back. Not enough blood is getting out of the ventricle and too much of it is regurgitating back in, so the ventricle is working far too hard, under internal pressures that are far too high—a recipe for lethal heart failure.

When Goldfarb is wheeled into the OR, he is met by an assistant surgeon, a physician's assistant, two anesthesiologists, and two OR nurses. The prep work takes about an hour. Goldfarb is anesthetized, shaved, and painted almost head to toe with bright red antiseptic; various monitoring leads and cuffs are affixed around his body, breathing and imaging tubes pushed down his throat, a flow monitoring catheter is threaded through the jugular vein into his heart, and a urinary catheter into his bladder. He is wrapped with yards and yards of sterile tape and gauze; his eyes are taped shut.

Before starting the surgery, the team must create a "sterile field," an invisible space surrounding the operating table. (Invisible, but known to everyone except me, the first time I was in an OR. I unwittingly started walking toward the edge of the field and was almost tackled by the head cardiac nurse, Flora Wang.) Within the field, "Surgeon's Rules" apply. No one may enter without first scrubbing hands and arms in a deep tub of antiseptic soap, and donning a long-sleeved, floor-length sterile surgical gown and sterile wrist-covering surgical gloves. All instruments, monitoring leads, and tubes that pass through the field must be sterile. At one point in the surgery, the physician's assistant, Debbie Savarese, brushed against a table outside the field. She immediately turned and raised her arms, and the nurse pulled off the surgical gown and helped her into a new one—just that slight brush was contaminating.

Goldfarb himself must be sterilized. A sterile plastic sheet is laid across his body and pressed down until it sticks like a second skin—the incision will be through the sheet. His entire body, including his face, is completely encased in sterile paper sheeting and dozens of blue OR towels. Anyone walking into the OR at that point would see only a mound of blue cloth, with an open, flesh-colored, plastic-covered strip about two feet long and six inches wide at the apex of the mound. The "scrub" nurse, who will work inside the field, rolls the instrument array—which she had arranged within a mini sterile field of its own—to the foot of the operating table and takes up her position on the right side. A plastic sterile sheet is raised behind Goldfarb's head. The sterile field is in place. Not everyone works inside the field. The anesthesiologists can operate all their monitoring and infusion equipment from behind the sheet, and do not gown. Flora Wang, who is serving as the "circulating" nurse that day, also stays outside the field. I am positioned with the anesthesiologists, standing on a low stool so I can see over the sheet directly down into Goldfarb's chest.

Raising the sheet palpably changes the tone in the room, like the pivotal rite in a religious ceremony. I've seen some noncardiac surgeries that were almost rowdy—loud rock music, locker-room jokes flying. But not in cardiac ORs. Some surgeons are notably more talkative than others, but once the sheet is up, the intense concentration imparts a note almost of solemnity. Mauricio Garrido, the assistant surgeon, has told me that cardiac surgery is one of the few procedures in which you are aware, at every moment, that your patient is at risk of sudden death; even simple mistakes can kill. Or as another surgeon, Allan Stewart, put it, "In heart surgery, the complications come at you very fast."

Smith arrives a few minutes later, quickly scrubs and gowns, and takes the lead surgeon's place on the right side of the table. Both he and Garrido wear bright headlamps and goggles with a jeweler's eyepiece for each eye. Garrido is the senior cardiac surgery resident, a fully qualified surgeon, who is completing two years of advanced training in heart and lung surgery. Normally, assistants open the chest, and Garrido has opened hundreds. But Goldfarb's opening poses special challenges, so Smith will lead it. The old bypass scar tissue in Goldfarb's chest has glued his heart to his chest wall, and the kind of saw used in a normal opening could wreak havoc. Even worse, one of the old bypasses—a vein graft that carries blood around a blocked coronary artery—snakes back and forth beneath the breastbone, or sternum, but Smith isn't completely sure of its location, so he has to be extra cautious.

Garrido makes the initial chest incision, using an electric scalpel that singes the flesh as it cuts—much as Western heroes cauterized their bullet wounds with branding irons. The smell of barbecued meat wafts through the room. Smith then goes to work on the sternum, using a small-bladed circular saw, working slowly, from the top down, with increasingly delicate strokes as he gets closer to the chest cavity.

When the sternum is finally split through, he and Garrido cautiously spread the halves a few inches apart and expose the solid mass of scar tissue. The two begin to "make a plane," separating the heart from the chest wall by cutting laterally along the inside of the wall. They cut from either side in tiny eighth-inch strokes, one of them bracing the chest as the other cuts. At one point, Smith takes two grapples, with blunt, rounded, claws, and hooks them under the chest wall. Then, neck muscles bulging, he leans back with his full weight to pull up his side of the chest to give Garrido a better working view. Garrido cuts for a while, then takes the grapples and does the same for Smith. As they gain separation, they insert a metal jack, or "retractor," and ratchet the sternum wide open—it looks slow and smooth, but I can feel the violent stretching and bending of the chest bones.

Making the plane takes almost two hours. During all that time, Smith and Garrido almost never speak, and take no breaks. Smith stretches his neck exactly twice, each time almost guiltily, suddenly arching his head back and flexing his shoulders in a one-second spasm. And they never deviate from the tedious rhythm of cautious, one-eighth-inch scalpel cuts.

There is a fleeting crisis. As they are almost finishing their plane, the anesthesiologist, Mark Heath, who is watching the EKG readout, says "Fib!" It's not loud, but it's sharp. I get out of the way: Goldfarb has fibrillated—instead of beating in rhythm, his heart muscle fibers are fluttering in aimless confusion. There is a flurry of motion: Wang sprints to the front to hand Smith electrical paddles from a defibrillating machine. A jolt from the paddles, the heart jerks, quivers, and resumes beating. Smith watches it for a few seconds, then he and Garrido resume their work.

Except for a couple of terse commands from Smith, no one has said anything. I had moved off to the side by the blood-bypass machine, and Allison Cohen, the bypass technician, or "perfusionist," said to me with a smile, "Well, that was mildly exciting." Her face was flushed and the smile looked nervous, but I assumed she really meant "mildly," for that was my impression. I had clearly seen an "event," but the team had moved quickly—I guessed the elapsed time at only twenty seconds or so. There was no shouting, and it all felt very controlled.

Later, I asked Smith. "Mildly exciting?" he said, "—no, that was *frightening*." Yes, your heart can stop for brief periods, he explained, but with a valve like Goldfarb's, it is very dangerous. The calcification on Goldfarb's valve stiffened it and made it hard to open. "My hands aren't strong enough to squeeze the ventricle and force open that valve," he said, "and the ventricle was still filling with blood. Another few seconds, it would have started to swell like a balloon, and nothing kills heart cells faster. We were, maybe, thirty seconds away from a fifty-fifty mortality situation. The bypass wasn't set up yet, so if the defibrillator hadn't worked right away, I would have had to crash on bypass through the groin. We had the equipment in place to do that, but it's a bloody, dangerous procedure, one that you really want to avoid."

How frightening? I asked. Once a week frightening? Once a year? Smith thought a bit—"About once a month." I asked why it had happened. "I don't know," he said. "It doesn't happen often—although we're always prepared for it—and it's hard to trace to specifics." Making the plane, he went on, required a long period of cutting around the pericardium, the sheath that encases the heart; conceivably, that could have disrupted the heart's electrical signals. But there was no way of knowing for sure.

When their "plane" is finally in place, Smith and Garrido prepare Goldfarb's heart for surgery. They slice open the pericardial sac and tie it back to expose the beating heart muscle, sequester chest arteries and lungs with a few large sutures, then insert the large tubes, or "cannulae," that will connect Goldfarb to the bypass machine—one is placed in the right atrium to intercept venous blood and shunt it to the machine, and a second is plugged into the aorta, to bring freshened blood back to Goldfarb. A second, smaller set of cannulae is placed in the aorta. After Goldfarb goes on the bypass machine, they will deliver "cardioplegia" into the coronary arteries to shut down the heart's beating and protect the myocardial cells. As the cannulae are being placed, Heath starts heparin infusions to prevent clotting during the surgery. When Goldfarb's clotting time registers about five times longer than normal, it is safe to go "on-pump."

Going on a bypass machine is routine in the sense that it takes place throughout the world literally thousands of times a day, but is never standard, especially if, as in Goldfarb's case, there is the danger of a sudden backup of blood. For almost ten minutes, Smith and Cohen go through a delicate series of maneuvers, easing open the bypass cannulae, while they alternately fill and drain the heart, until it is completely empty and circulation is under the control of the machine. Smith announces "Cross-clamp" and applies a large clamp that completely shuts off the aorta just below the bypass cannula. Cohen starts the cardioplegia, and Goldfarb's heart jitters to a stop. She flips a switch to turn on a blood-cooling device to lower Goldfarb's body temperature, which reduces the risk of prolonged surgery. Heath turns off the ventilator, or breathing pump, and Goldfarb's lungs deflate. For the duration of the operation, the bypass machine will detour Goldfarb's blood around his heart and lungs, process it through a series of vertical spinning cylinders where it will be mixed with air, and pump it back into the aorta.

It is now more than three hours into the operation, and the valve replacement can finally get under way. Smith makes an incision at the base of the aorta to expose the aortic valve. He probes the thick encrustations of calcium, then like plumbers repairing an old pipe fitting, he and Garrido chip away calcium, carefully removing any stray pieces—floating calcium debris could trigger a stroke. They then slice out the three valve leaflets and trim back the white, rubbery ring that they sit on, leaving just enough to anchor the new valve.

Goldfarb had chosen a replacement valve derived from a cow. It won't last as long as a purely mechanical model, but avoids the necessity of a lifelong anticlotting regimen. For a flat, firm valve placement, the suturing must be straight and kink-free, and Smith and Garrido take elaborate precautions against tangles. They space twelve separate sutures, in alternating blue and white, around the rim of the empty valve opening, each one pulled through the rim and folded back on the towels in a double strand.

As they finish a set of four, they cover it with another towel. Both ends of each suture are then stitched through the sewing ring around the outside of the valve. Smith carefully pushes the valve down the columns of sutures into the valve opening and presses it firmly in place—it is by that point only partly visible. He takes each suture pair, holds it up for the nurse to clip off the needles, and, his fingers a blur, ties a triple square knot that slides down tightly to the top of the valve ring. When he finishes, Garrido sprays away accumulated blood, while Smith uses a probe for a long, careful, inspection of each of the attachment points. The two then reseal the aorta with two layers of closely spaced, evenly slanted continuous stitching, much like that on the outside of a moccasin.

Cohen has already started warming the bypass blood, and as Goldfarb's temperature rises back to normal, they ease him off bypass—essentially reversing the process of going on-pump. Cohen washes out the cardioplegia and flushes warm blood through the coronary arteries. Goldfarb's heart immediately starts to quiver. Smith eases up on the aortic cross-clamp, while Cohen slowly closes off the venous cannula, redirecting blood back into the heart. Heath restarts the ventilator, and Smith opens a small tube he prepositioned in the heart to bubble out accumulated air. As soon as Goldfarb's heart fills with blood, it jerks back to life, beats strongly for a few minutes, then starts jumping erratically, registering rounded, somewhat incoherent lines on the EKG. Smith applies pacing wires, and the EKG readings quickly shift into the evenly spaced, sharply pointed profile of a normal heartbeat. Cohen turns off the bypass, and Heath injects a heparin antidote that almost instantly drops Goldfarb's clotting time back to normal.

For several minutes everyone focuses on the echocardiogram image of the new valve, as Heath manipulates the receptor in Goldfarb's throat to show it from different angles. It's clearly a good valve, opening and closing smoothly and tightly. Smith makes one last inspection of the aortic stitches, then he and Garrido start extracting the bypass tubing and closing the incisions. Remarkably, Goldfarb has not needed a transfusion. Blood accumulating in his chest cavity has been siphoned out to the bypass machine, where it has been cleaned and added to the bypass volume. In a good heart center, most patients lose very little blood.

Garrido and Savarese handle the cleanup and chest closing, although Smith checks on their progress from time to time. It takes about an hour—taking out the temporary sutures, removing the multiple absorbent cloths and towels in the chest cavity (especially checking that no blood-soaked, bunched-up cloths are jammed beneath Goldfarb's heart), installing pacing wires and a drainage tube through Goldfarb's chest, reinspecting each stitching site.

Finally, Garrido removes the chest retractor and starts placing a row of heavy stainless steel sternal sutures, pushing them up from under the sternum on each side, and twisting them closed at the top. When they are all in place, Goldfarb's chest still gapes open by several inches. Using a heavy pliers, and starting from the bottom, Garrido tightens each twist, slowly tractoring the two sides of Goldfarb's chest back together. Garrido is stocky and strongly built, but Goldfarb is a big man: it takes about ten minutes and a half dozen passes to get a tight closure. The last step is to stitch shut the chest flesh over the sternum. The stitching is in several layers, with Garrido and Savarese each working from a different end of the incision to the middle. All of the stitches are subcutaneous, so when I saw Goldfarb a few days later, his chest showed only a narrow red line with no stitch markings. The flesh stitches will degrade and be absorbed over several weeks, but the sternal sutures are there for life.

By the time the stitching is finished, the transport team has arrived from the ICU. Shifting dead weight like Goldfarb's from the operating table to a gurney would be tricky under any circumstances, but is made doubly so by the drips, tubes, wires, and machinery still attached to his body. Between the transport team and the OR team, there are eight people in the room. They all take positions around Goldfarb and with a "One-two-three-lift!" move him onto the gurney. In the ICU, Goldfarb will be settled in a bed, attached to a range of monitors to track his circulation, heart performance, and other vital functions, and checked for any signs of bleeding or excess drainage. A painkilling drip will be attached to his chest; when he is stable and his bleeding under control, he will slowly be awakened from the anesthesia. It is well past noon when the gurney leaves the OR, some five hours after Goldfarb's arrival. My back and legs are painfully stiff from the hours of standing, but Garrido and Savarese have one, and possibly two, more operations to go. There is time for a bathroom break and a quick snack before getting back to work.

Goldfarb was released from the ICU after the standard two days. The next stop was a "step-down" unit, roughly the same as a normal hospital floor, but with double the nursing ratio. I visited him there on "POD 4," or the fourth postoperative day. He was sitting in a chair by the bed, eating lunch. He was clearly weak, but compared to my last image—mostly of a bloody hole atop a mound of blue towels—"weak" looked pretty good. Pain was not much of a problem, he reported, although his chest was stiff and sore. His Parkinson's medication hadn't been resumed right away, so his hand tremor had returned, but was already getting better. I asked about his breathing. He said, "Before the surgery, I couldn't walk a hundred yards. I think I could walk around the block right now." And he was in fact already walking regularly on the floor and doing breathing exercises. This was a Thursday; he expected to move that day or the next to a regular floor. Assuming no setbacks, he would be discharged the next Monday to his daughter's apartment in New York, where he would stay until he could return to Florida.

I stayed for about a half hour. We talked mostly about the pharmacy business: he explained how the government was destroying neighborhood druggists by pushing Medicare clients into mail-order programs. But his manner was relaxed and smiling, belying his words. The surgery was over, he was going to be fine, and he was able to sit and talk about business. He looked like a happy man.

I called his daughter's apartment about three weeks later to see how he was doing. A booming male voice answered. I said, "Mr. Goldfarb?" He sounded nothing like the Mr. Goldfarb I had met before the surgery. Yes, it was Mr. Goldfarb, and he was doing spectacularly well. "I'll be grateful forever to Dr. Smith for fixing my valve," he said, "but the nutritionist at the hospital changed my life." All patients meet with a nutritionist before they leave the hospital; she told him she had just visited a man his age who had not managed his diabetes and was now a quadruple amputee. "She scared the hell out of me," Goldfarb said. "I've never paid attention to my diabetes. I never checked my glucose, I took the same medication every day, and I ate what I felt like." Since the surgery, he had lost 23 pounds and was planning to keep it off. He was tracking his glucose religiously, and his cholestrol was down to 152. He was walking around his daughter's neighborhood several times a day. Even his sciatica was gone! "I've been given a second chance," he said. "Actually, it's your third,'" I said. He laughed, "You're right. It's my third. But it's finally gotten through to me, and I'm going to make the most of it."

The total cost of Goldfarb's surgery, including a reasonable allowance for aftercare, was about $65,000. But if the cost is measured per "quality year" of life gained for patients like Goldfarb, it would be well under $10,000. Most economists say that's a bargain, although many still worry about its affordability. We will come back to the question of affordability in the last chapter. But the ability even to perform procedures like Mr. Goldfarb's didn't just happen. It is the consequence of a purposeful, highly focused, public-private research effort that stretches back a half century and beyond.

Chapter 2

A VERY SHORT HISTORY OF HEART SURGERY

Cave paintings from 20,000 years ago show game animals with spears sticking out of unmistakably drawn hearts. They may have been the first graphic textbooks—if you want to kill a big animal, *that's* where you stab it.

Chinese physicians were writing of the diagnostic implications of patient pulse rates almost 5,000 years ago, and may have guessed that blood circulates. In the West, the two millennia from the Greeks to the European Enlightenment were dominated by Hippocrates' theory of four "humors," in which the heart was the source of "vital heat" and blood was more often associated with the liver. Diligent anatomists like Aristotle, Galen, and Avicenna worked out the heart's internal structures, and had a reasonable understanding of diastolic and systolic blood pressures, the functioning of the valves, and much else. Leonardo da Vinci made gorgeous drawings of the human heart and its major valves in the late fifteenth century, and Andreas Vesalius, a mid-sixteenth-century prosecutor in Padua, and an enthusiastic autopsist, carried cardiac anatomy to near-modern levels of precision.

But it was left to the seventeenth-century Englishman William Harvey to elucidate how all that apparatus really worked, much as his great contemporary Galileo did for astronomy and physics. Harvey conducted the experiments that proved the existence of the capillaries, the circulation of the blood, the direction of its flow, the heart-lung cycle, the action of the heartbeat, the role of the ventricle, and much else—all of which the microscopists resoundingly confirmed within a few decades of his first announcements.

At first, the more clinicians learned about the heart, the more they were convinced it was an untouchable organ. During the Napoleonic wars, however, a few adventurous surgeons figured out that when blood or pus from an injury swelled the pericardium (the sheath around the heart) and cut off circulation, they could often cure a patient by making a drainage incision. But they were still careful not to touch the heart itself. By the mid-nineteenth century, however, accumulating autopsy evidence of scars on the hearts of fighting men suggested that the heart might be able to recover from a wound. Animal experiments demonstrated the feasibility of suturing wounds in the heart by the 1880s.

The first successful human heart operation took place in 1896 in Frankfurt, on a young man who had been stabbed in a brawl. The surgeon opened the pericardium to drain suppurative fluids, then closed a 1.5 cm wound of the right ventricle. The man was reported still alive ten years later. The first heart operation in the United States was performed in 1902 on a kitchen table in an Alabama "negro cabin." The patient was a thirteen-year-old boy who had been stabbed multiple times in the chest. The procedure was much like that in Frankfurt, with a Dr. Luther Hill of Montgomery performing the surgery. Hill pierced and drained a bloody buildup in the pericardium, after which the boy's pulse noticeably improved, and then he closed a three-eighths-inch stab wound in the heart, packing it, as in Frankfurt, with iodine-soaked gauze to ward off infection. The boy apparently recovered.

The carnage of the First World War brought more impromptu experiments. Although survival rates were very poor, interest kept rising. During the intrawar years, researchers in widely disparate fields began to assemble the technological matrix for reliable cardiac surgical interventions—including the beginnings of dye-based X-ray angiography (injecting X-ray-reflective dye into the heart to locate blockages), rapid strides in both anesthesia and antisepsis, and the discovery of heparin to reduce clotting and of antibiotics to combat infections. The electrical patterns of the heartbeat were being deciphered, and work had commenced on electric pacemakers. Animal experimenters were also starting to understand how resilient the heart is. In one experiment, researchers completely drained a dog's blood from its body, waited for several minutes, then reinfused the blood and were amazed to see the heart restart. During World War II, surgeons had some success in removing projectiles from soldiers' hearts, and cardiology began to emerge as a recognized medical specialty.

Research interest in cardiac medicine was driven by growing alarm over the steady increase in cardiovascular death rates. As the wealthiest people in history, Americans were eating more and more richly, were more likely to have sedentary jobs, and, with the spread of the automobile, did much less walking. By the 1950s, cardiovascular disease was an epidemic of crisis proportions, accounting for more than half of all American deaths.

The technology of cardiac surgery began to assume its current shape through the 1950s and 1960s. Thomas J. Watson, Jr., the chairman of IBM, made a personal project of financing and developing the heart-lung bypass machine, based on a prototype that a surgeon, John Gibbons, had built in 1937. Gibbons performed the first successful operation on a human with the assistance of the bypass machine in 1953. He repaired an atrial septal defect, a hole in the internal wall separating the left and right atria; the machine was built by IBM.

The bypass machine made "direct-vision" heart surgery possible for the first time. With the heart off-line, a surgeon could open it, inspect the problem, and often repair it. Prior to the bypass machine, surgeons were limited to operations that could be performed entirely outside the heart, like suturing wounds, or ones that they could do solely by feel—a balky mitral valve could sometimes be opened by making a tiny incision, sticking in a finger, feeling for the valve, and pushing it open. The first widely adopted bypass-machine protocols were established in a famous series of operations by John Kirklin, at the Mayo Clinic in 1955.

Enthusiasm for on-pump—bypass-machine—surgery

was dampened as it became clear that the machine itself could cause serious cardiovascular and cerebral complications. Over time, however, as machine-associated complications were brought down to acceptable levels, the heart-lung bypass machine revolutionized cardiac surgery. As valve replacement became a practical alternative in the 1960s, there was a vast florescence of replacement-valve designs, including valves from human cadavers; equine, bovine, and porcine valves; and dozens of mechanical valves. An early ball-and-cage aortic valve worked reasonably well, but clicked open and shut so loudly that it embarrassed its users.

The most consequential development of the period, however, was the coronary artery bypass graft, or CABG, universally pronounced "cabbage." Occlusions of the coronaries, the arteries that supply blood to the heart, were identified in the nineteenth century. The occlusive material—calcium, cholesterol, microemboli and other cell detritus—is now known to be a partial correlate of rich diets and minimal exercise. Doctors had long understood the connection between coronary occlusions and angina pain. Symptomatic treatments included amyl nitrate, a vascular relaxant, and in the 1920s and 1930s, thyroid removal. (Excising the thyroid lowered adrenaline production so the heart reacted less quickly to stimuli. Quick ramp-ups in cardiac output often precipitated angina attacks. The underlying occlusion was unaffected.)

Since coronary arteries are usually on the outside of the heart, surgeons could work on them even before the development of the bypass machine. The intrawar years saw multiple attempts at opening and cleaning occluded coronaries, with little success. In the 1940s, however, surgeons hit upon the idea of simply implanting one end of a mammary artery directly into the heart. Remarkably, instead of just creating a trapped pool of blood, the implanted artery gradually generated a rich network of new blood vessels within the myocardium. The first mammary implant was performed on a human in 1950 and was a complete success. Three years later, the patient, who had been completely debilitated before the operation, was taking ten-mile hikes. As the technique spread, it appeared that some 70 to 80 percent of surviving patients experienced substantial revascularization within eighteen months or so of the operation. About one in three patients died from the operation, however, which was fairly typical of the heart surgery of the time.

The modern CABG was developed at the Cleveland Clinic in the 1960s, primarily by the Argentinean surgeon René Favaloro, working closely with Frank Sones, a key contributor to modern cardiac angiography. Favaloro performed an unusually successful series of mammary artery implants in 1964, but was bent on finding more direct methods with more immediate results. He performed the first successful CABG on a human in 1967. The procedure entailed excising a vein from the patient's leg, grafting one end to the diseased coronary artery just below the occlusion and the other end to the aorta. The occlusion was thereby "bypassed" and that portion of the heart once again received a full blood supply. By the following year, Favaloro had performed 171 bypasses with a mortality rate of only 5 percent—at first provoking wide disbelief among his contemporaries.

Having firmly demonstrated the effectiveness of the CABG against angina, the next year Favaloro showed that the same operation, performed within six hours of a heart attack, had a substantial effect in preserving heart muscle. By the end of the year, he had also performed the first double bypass. In the course of his work, Favaloro also established the center-line sternotomy, or breastbone incision, as the standard mode of surgical access, made a number of contributions to improving the bypass machine, and invented the chest retractor. Forty years later, most cardiac surgeons still execute CABGs more or less the way Favaloro did.

By 1970, Favaloro's breakthroughs had triggered the explosive growth of a new medical industry. There were 60,000 CABG operations in the United States in 1975, and 250,000 in 1985. By the early 1990s, when annual CABG numbers hovered around 350,000, almost every medium-sized city in the country could boast of an open-heart surgery center. Outstanding centers, like those of the great surgeons and bitter rivals Denton Cooley and Michael DeBakey in Houston, became heart surgery Meccas, drawing patients from all over the world. Despite its extraordinary invasiveness and high costs, the CABG became almost fashionable.

The explosion of investment in cardiac intervention had implications far beyond the operating table—rapid-response interventions, tools and techniques to increase diagnostic precision and speed, specialized cardiac care units, better methods of heart protection during surgery, and a steady expansion of the numbers of ailments and patients within reach of the cardiac treatment web. As surgical morbidity and mortality rates dropped to levels that had been unimaginable a decade or so before, patient demographics shifted rapidly to older and riskier patients. Only 4 percent of today's CABG patients would have been eligible for the surgery under the original guidelines. Mortality rates jumped sharply at first, but quickly settled back to previous levels. One consequence of removing CABG age limits was that women, who tend to contract cardiovascular disease later than men, entered the patient pool in large numbers. By the 1980s, transplant technology, as well, was on the verge of entering the mainstream.

Especially in its high-growth days, the momentum behind CABGs led to substantial overuse, much as may be happening today with stents. (Stents are tiny metal scaffolds that are used to prop open a blocked artery; they are delivered with a catheter inserted through an artery, so they don't require surgery.) Several long-term randomized studies from the late 1970s and 1980s, however, clearly demonstrated the mortality benefits of the CABG for higher-risk patients—those with either multiple occluded vessels or occlusions in the major arteries of the left ventricle. The CABG also clearly relieved symptoms of severe angina, but with little mortality benefit.

The public health impact from the massive new investment in heart disease infrastructure was substantial. One statistic captures it all. Between 1970 and 1995, heart attack hospitalizations per 100,000 Americans dropped from 530 to 490, about a 7.5 percent decline. Over the same period, the heart attack *death rate* per 100,000 dropped from 256 to only 70, a 72.8 percent decrease. Stripping out all other factors that might account for the change in heart attack death rates, there is a near-consensus that as much as 70 percent of it was the result of better medical interventions. Just since the mid-1970s, total federal investment in cardiovascular research and treatment infrastructure exceeds $30 billion.

The rapid-growth phase of cardiac surgery ended sometime in the mid-1990s, and the profession began to acquire some of the hallmarks of what stock analysts might call a "maturing" business. But that is another story, to which we will return in Chapter 8.

Chapter 3

ARTISANS
AT WORK

I GLIMPSED THE REWARDS OF BEING A HEART SUR-
geon while accompanying Craig Smith and Mike Argenziano on postoperative patient rounds. Argenziano, at
thirty-nine, is one of the younger surgeons, four years out
of the division's residency program. He is tall, bluff, and
cheerful, and clearly enjoys bantering with the patients.
On his rounds, Smith is characteristically reserved, but
concerned and personal—asking focused, careful questions with a lot of touching. For each of them, however,
the visits were triumphal processions, choruses of cheers—
"I thank you from the bottom of my heart, Dr. Smith!"
"You went above and beyond the call of duty, Dr. Argenziano!" ("No, I didn't," Argenziano smiles, "I just did
what you paid me for.")

At a careers meeting with Columbia medical students,
Eric Rose, the chairman of the Department of Surgery, and
a cardiothoracic surgeon himself, suggested that students
who enjoyed "fixing problems" should consider going into

surgery. Those who naturally preferred "intellectualizing" problems ("nothing wrong with that," he insisted) should go into medicine. Smith told the same group the sad tale of a brilliant medical school friend who had gone into medical practice and now sees only "an endless stream of patients with obesity, diabetes, and hypertension." A special attraction of heart surgery, compared to, say, cancer surgery is that the results are usually quite clear-cut. After Smith replaced Mr. Goldfarb's aortic valve, for example, you could see it smoothly opening and closing on the echo screen—whatever Goldfarb's health worries, he could cross that valve off the list. Orthopedic surgery has a similar practical, mechanical, flavor, but isn't accompanied by the constant refrain of "Thank you, doctor, you saved my life."

There are fourteen full-time surgeons, called "attendings," in the cardiothoracic division. Although they all can work with any of the division's patients, there is de facto specialization. Five of them, including Smith, account for almost all the adult cardiac surgery, three for almost all the pediatric surgery, while one concentrates on pacemakers and defibrillators. There is also a thoracic section with five surgeons devoted almost exclusively to lung surgery.*

---

*Training for "cardiothoracic" surgery entails working on both heart and lungs, since they are properly viewed as a unified respiratory/circulatory system. The recent trend has been to specialize in one or the other after training, and the accreditation authorities are now moving to begin the specialization from the very start of training. I focus almost exclusively on the cardiac side, in part because the practices are really quite different—lung surgeons, for example, are much more involved with cancers—and I decided it was too much to absorb. In addition, as one of the lung surgeons conceded, although the lung is amazingly complex, it is the much less glamorous organ.

Since transplants are a young man's game, requiring heroic tolerance for sleep deprivation, the younger attendings in both the cardiac and thoracic sections take turns on transplant duty. The surgeons are assisted by four cardiothoracic surgical trainees, dubbed "residents" or "fellows," all of them qualified general surgeons spending two years learning the cardiothoracic specialty. And there is typically a handful of "superfellows," former residents who have completed their training but who have chosen to extend their residencies, perhaps to complete promising research projects, or to resolve citizenship issues. Finally, there are a half dozen or so research fellows supporting the division's various research initiatives—most of them young doctors taking a break from general surgical training in the hope of improving their chances of qualifying for a top cardiothoracic program.

Heart surgeons are reputed to be fiercely competitive, with giant egos—the working atmosphere at another New York hospital was described to me as "cutthroat"—and I supposed that would be especially so in a high-profile place like Columbia. I was surprised, therefore, at the easy collegiality that prevailed at the first division meetings I attended. The meetings are large ones, usually about thirty-plus people—the attendings, the residents, some of the research fellows, most of the perfusionists, usually with doctors from affiliated heart hospitals sitting in via video-conferencing feed. There was little sense of hierarchy. The attendings did most of the talking, but the residents participated freely, as did Linda Mongero, the director of the perfusionists, who is neither a doctor nor even officially part of the division. Smith did not sit at the head of the table or visibly run the meeting, although when he summarized the discussion, it was usually a signal to move on.

That collegial operating mode, it turns out, is highly valued throughout the division. Indeed, when I spoke to people, it was often one of the first things they mentioned. Mehmet Oz, who along with Smith is one of the two senior adult cardiac surgeons, said, "This is a very tough place, but it's a happy place to work. We all care a lot about each other." It is a style that apparently dates back to the late Keith Reemtsma, a revered, long-serving surgery department chairman (and also the real-life model for the Hawkeye character in *M*A*S*H*); and it has been carried on by Smith and by Rose, Smith's predecessor as cardiothoracic chief. "Keith could never tolerate interpersonal bullshit," says Oz. "Craig is like that too, and Eric is like that. When I was a young attending, at times I was too tough, and Eric would pull me in. He'd say, it's just not how we do business—do you want to be mad, or do you want to solve the problem?"

The group's problem-solving skills are impressive. I kept notes on two potentially rancorous discussions—one related to selecting final candidates for a new residency class, and the other involved allocating OR time when the rooms are backed up, which directly affects attendings' earnings. What struck me was not that they reached reasonable resolutions, but that throughout the discussions, positions were framed in the strongest tones—phrases such as "I completely disagree with you" were tossed around freely—but without raised voices, reddened faces, or banged fists. In effect, disagreements were treated as

awkward facts, perhaps not unlike a poor surgical outcome. They were unfortunate but had to be discussed
frankly and civilly, and managed without animosity.

Allan Stewart, the youngest attending, just a year out of
his residency, told me that the division's problem-solving
facility was "one of the reasons I wanted to work here.
It's not that we're all best friends. But if you have an issue,
you discuss it, all the strong personalities come out, and at
the end of the day you have an answer—whether it's an
answer you like or don't like. Craig is a big factor in making that work, because he never exerts muscle. You never
hear him say, 'It has to be this way because I'm chief!' "

Jack Shanewise, chief of the cardiothoracic anesthesiology section, is a relative newcomer to Columbia and has
worked at a number of other institutions. He remarked to
me on the very high quality of the Columbia surgeons.
The typical surgical unit, he said, has its stars and weak
sisters. "But that's not true here," he told me. "*All* of them
are very good. That's rare." Another anesthesiologist,
Johanna Schwarzenberger, who has trained and worked
throughout both the United States and Europe, agreed
with Shanewise. The division's surgeons are the best she's
ever worked with, she says, but suggests that the style of
interaction is part of the reason. "There is a constant conversation at Columbia," she says. "Every decision is ques-
tioned, all the time. It's a unique place."

Smith's decade-plus tenure as chief has left its own
stamp. His professional personality is austere to the point
of frostiness. Junior residents find him intimidating—
impatient with their shortcomings and very sparing of
praise; and in the monthly reviews of problem cases—the

"Morbidity and Mortality" meetings—Smith is always the most critical. People put up with it, not because he's chief, but because they know he is even harder on himself. He's "sparse on compliments," Oz smiles, but "ruthless in self-criticism." Mauricio Garrido told me, "Smith was a big reason I wanted to come here. Technically, he's awesome, but the character issues were more important—his way of leading, his brutal honesty." Mike Bowdish, the junior resident when I started my research, after recounting an especially painful day under Smith's unforgiving eye, ended by saying, "But he's the finest surgeon I've ever met. There are others as good technically, but Smith is so ethical." When I pushed him to explain "ethical" he talked about Smith's honesty, his scrupulousness in visiting his patients, his sense of responsibility for the outcomes. Bill Clinton also made a special point of Smith's "values" in his presentation of Smith's 2007 Heart Association award—besides being a fine doctor, he said, Smith is "a good man." Smith's position as chief is reinforced by the fact that, instead of pushing himself as the division's star, he has helped each of the younger attendings to develop a high-profile specialty of his own—Argenziano in minimally invasive techniques, Stewart in aortic surgery, and Yoshifumi Naka in transplants and heart-assist devices.*

Finally, the phenomenon of Mehmet Oz deserves a note of its own. Oz's family immigrated from Turkey a few

---

*At dinner with a doctor friend from another Columbia division, he groused about the way his division split up fee income. I mentioned that in Cardiothoracic Smith made the splits himself. He said, "Sure. But everybody knows he's so fair." Characteristically, Smith is not Cardiothoracic's highest-paid surgeon.

years before he was born. His father, now a heart surgeon in Delaware, came from a dirt-poor but fiercely self-improving peasant family—every one of the children became a college professor. His mother was from one of the wealthiest families in Turkey; they were immigrants from Circassia who became Istanbul business tycoons. When Oz was a kid, he alternated summers between his father's and his mother's families—one summer living in a dirt-floor hut without running water or electricity, threshing wheat by hand, and the next in a mansion tended by a phalanx of servants. "I wasn't an outsider in either environment," he said. "I was an insider in both. To this day, it's made me a comfortable chameleon." His mother, he said, always gave him "uncritical love," while his father drove him. We were talking in his office early one morning in the spring. Oz had just returned from Turkey, where he had given a speech—"It was a big deal," he said, "on national television and so forth. There was a family party afterward, and I asked my father what he thought. He answered in Turkish, the same expression he always used, meaning 'There were deficiencies.' If I got a 98 in school instead of 100, he'd say, 'You'll never be a big man.'"

Oz was an outstanding student, and the first all-state football player at his high school. He played varsity football at Harvard, went to medical school at the University of Pennsylvania, and also got a business degree at Penn's Wharton School before coming to Columbia as a surgical resident. He has had three *New York Times* best-sellers, is a regular on *Oprah*, has had his own Discovery Channel series, and made a list of *People* magazine's "sexiest doctors." He is also active in New Jersey politics and a regular at the Davos World Economic Forum. His research interests span both standard medicine and alternative medicine—"integrative," as he calls it.

A few weeks after meeting with Oz, I was speaking with Henry Spotnitz, the vice chairman for research in the surgery department. We were talking about publishing requirements for academic surgeons—about three papers a year, which is high. I asked whether those rules applied to residents, given their insane work schedules. He said generally not. "Of course, when Mehmet Oz was a resident," he added, "he had fifty-five first-author papers." "I'm good at building systems that succeed," Oz had told me, "factories that publish papers, laboratories that work relatively simplistically. When I was captain of a team in sports, I was good at helping everyone else excel, because they helped me excel."

Oz is still close to his extended Turkish family, and he speaks warmly of his own family. His wife is an actress and producer; their four kids range from elementary-school age to early twenties. While we were talking, he was interrupted by a phone call about a relative who was stuck in the Frankfurt airport—whatever the confusion was, it took just a couple of calls to straighten out. Then he introduced me to a niece, a medical student in Istanbul, who was spending a season in his lab. A little later, I sat in on an initial meeting with his new crop of lab assistants. I counted twelve to fifteen young people, although there was considerable coming and going. Two of them were Columbia surgical residents, taking a residency break to sharpen their research skills, but the rest were medical students or headed to medical school, and drawn from all over the world—Eastern

Europe, Africa, Pakistan, Turkey—"kids with no inside track," he said. He opened the session by handing each new assistant a copy of Strunk and White's *Elements of Style*, the classic handbook of good writing. "*This* may be the most important book anyone ever gives you. Study it every day. No matter how smart you are, or how much you know about medicine, it will make no difference if you can't express yourselves effectively." I'm biased, of course, but I hoped they listened.

Virtuosos at Work

Columbia-Presbyterian's cardiothoracic division is a business—doctors see patients and perform operations, and are well paid for their work. But it is also part of a university. The attendings are all Columbia University faculty, explicitly charged with training a new generation of surgeons and advancing the boundaries of their profession. Although perfectly standard operations, like the plain-vanilla coronary artery bypass graft, or CABG, make up a good portion of their practice, a substantial number are virtuosic undertakings in which approaches and techniques are still in a state of flux. I skewed the procedures I observed toward the nonroutine end of the spectrum. A few cases give the flavor.

The first was a Smith specialty, a quintuple "beating heart," or "off-pump" CABG—without the heart-lung bypass machine, and with the use of arterial grafts instead of the normal leg-vein graft. The heart-lung machine has long been suspected as the source of the neurocognitive deficits that sometimes follow prolonged heart surgery. The unnatural machine pressures, and turbulence at cannula entry points, create a hailstorm of tiny fat globules, clots, and other detritus that are small enough to penetrate the brain's safety barrier and do real damage. Although tools and techniques for off-pump surgery have become available within the last decade, only a minority of surgeons are comfortable working with them. Similarly, leg veins are much weaker vessels than arteries—the fluid dynamics within arteries are much more demanding—and are a frequent source of bypass failure. Mammary arteries from the chest make much better bypass conduits, and bring their own blood supply besides. (The surgeon can just disconnect the downstream end and graft it to the target, while a vein graft has to be attached both to the target coronary artery and to the aorta, as a source of fresh blood.) But arteries are hard to work with—they're small and rubbery, and encased in multilayered sheathing. Although they are the graft of choice at Columbia-Presbyterian, most heart surgeons still stick with leg veins. A beating-heart quintuple CABG with primarily arterial grafts, therefore, is a bravura performance, although fairly standard for Smith.

I was surprised how much of the operation had to be devised on the fly. Two residents opened the chest and prepared a leg vein and two mammary arteries for the grafts. Smith was planning to use the left mammary artery for the left heart grafts, but it was too short. So he excised it from the chest, cut it into two segments, plugged those into the other chest artery to make a branching system with three outlets, and used that to repair three diseased coronary arteries on the front of the heart. Since the last two target grafts were on the back of the heart, Smith placed a suction-cup device on the bottom point of the heart, its "apex," so the resident could ratchet the heart up out of the chest and twist it backward to expose the two targets. (On the EKG, the heartbeat never wavered.) He cut the leg vein into a long segment and a short one, joined them to make a Y-shaped outlet, grafted the two outlets to the target coronary arteries, and then ran the long end up to the aorta. As he explained later, while imaging technology is good at locating blockages, the surgeon still has to see and touch the heart to know whether it's even possible to work off-pump,* how readily the coronaries can be bypassed, or the most efficient way to lay out the new plumbing.

The whole operation was yet another demonstration of the astonishing power of sustained concentration possessed by elite surgeons. Each of the grafts involved about twenty minutes of fiddly, fine-grained work—clamping and making slits in the source and the target vessels, all of them in slippery, wriggly motion, then joining the slits with almost invisible sutures to make a free-flowing, leak-proof junction. A normal craftsman, faced with a similar series of intense little tasks, would take a short break after each one—straighten up, stretch his back, have a sip of

---

*Coronary arteries are usually on the outside of the myocardium, which makes them easily accessible without opening the heart. Otherwise, as in virtually all valve work, the use of the heart-lung machine is unavoidable. And occasionally, some arteries in the back of the heart, next to the rear chest wall, can't be reached without going on-pump to drain the heart. Smith does about 70 percent of his bypasses off-pump, sometimes executing the first several off-pump, then using the pump for the last one or two.

coffee, walk around the room. Smith executed all five in
a bit less than an hour and a half, without pausing, and
without even lifting his head. When the patient is on the
table, his heart beating and exposed to the world, you
don't take coffee breaks.

A few days later, I watched Argenziano perform a minimally invasive repair of a mitral valve, the valve that sits
between the heart's left atrium, where blood flows in from
the lungs, and the left ventricle. While the aortic valve has
an elegantly simple design—a case study for the theory of
intelligent design—the mitral valve, just a few inches
away, is a nice counterdemonstration of evolutionary
making-do. With only two flaps instead of three, it's prone
to leakiness, and the flaps have to be supported by a complicated apparatus of muscles and tendons. The standard
mitral-valve therapy is replacement with a mechanical
valve, but techniques for mitral repair have been evolving
rapidly. Smith himself did much of the early work and,
Argenziano told me, made Columbia-Presbyterian a
"Mecca for repair." The repair is usually executed by trim-
ming the valve flaps and tightening the diameter of the
valve ring—straightforward enough in concept, but still
very much the province of experts. Done properly, however, a repaired valve promises longer, more trouble-free
operation than one from a manufacturer's shelf.

Combining mitral repair with minimally invasive
access, as Argenziano was doing, ratcheted up the degree
of difficulty. Minimally invasive techniques for extracting
gall bladders and the like caught on like wildfire in the
early 1990s, but are still controversial in heart surgery.
Smith points out that the original term was "minimal

access," but that was felt to have negative connotations. While smaller incisions conduce to faster healing, less infection, less buildup of scar tissue, and much better cosmetics, they also limit the surgeon's field of vision and require him to work at a greater distance from his target with specially adapted tools. It takes a lot of practice to get comfortable with the methods, and operations generally take longer, which may entail more time on bypass. But patients love them—the vanity-driven urge to avoid chest scars is extraordinary, even among people who should be beyond caring. Argenziano had just finished his residency when Smith assigned him to develop Columbia-Presbyterian's minimally invasive program—to master the techniques and establish best practices. He is now the division's minimally invasive guru and has made a number of practice contributions in his own right.

For a minimally invasive mitral repair, the surgeon makes a six-inch incision between two ribs on the right side of the chest. The ribs are spread open with a small retractor, but not broken, and the right lung is deflated to expose the heart, opening a clear path to the mitral. With such a small working space, placing the bypass cannulae is a feat in itself, and Argenziano has pioneered a procedure of turning the heart several centimeters to facilitate the placing of the aortic cannula. The venous cannula is usually placed in a leg vein to reduce the tubing in the mitral access space. Argenziano is a tall man with large hands. Although the table was tilted to one side to facilitate right chest access, he still had to crouch during much of the surgery and, he told me later, always scrapes his hands raw on the retractor. Tying good knots at a distance is another challenge—there are a number of knot-placing tools available, but Argenziano, like most surgeons, prefers to feel the tension with his fingers.

The valve was repaired without mishap, the echo showed it working as it should, and I was later told the patient was delighted with her quick recovery time. But I was impressed with the trickiness of the approach. Surgeons shouldn't attempt minimally invasive mitrals, Argenziano said, unless "you've done so many that you can do them blindfolded, because that's almost what it's like." Argenziano's own safety record with the techniques is as at least as good as the standard for open-chest procedures, but he is selective in his patients and still turns down a majority of those who request them.

My third example, a *pièce de résistance*, was an "arterial switch." Birth defects account for quite a high proportion of cardiac surgery. At Columbia-Presbyterian, "congenital" heart surgery is the preserve of the pediatric section, since the great majority of cases, and all the most challenging ones, are pediatric. (Adult congenital patients necessarily have milder diseases, or they would not have survived.) The arterial switch is an operation to repair a cataclysmic heart malformation in newborns, known as "transposition of the great vessels" (TGV), in which the pulmonary artery and the aorta are misconnected—the aorta delivers blood into the lungs while the pulmonary artery dumps venous blood into the arterial system.

Separating a TGV baby from the umbilical cord would be a fast death sentence, except that TGV is usually accompanied by other malformations that allow blood to slosh back and forth between the left and right ventricles.

In the more extreme cases, the left and right ventricle are merged into a single chamber—in effect, both the lungs and the arterial system are getting blood that is half-oxygenated. If the admixture between the chambers is low, the baby will present as an oxygen-starved "blue baby" (which can also result from a variety of other congenital problems). But sometimes the mixing is rich enough that the baby appears perfectly normal. People born with TGV occasionally survive into adulthood, but if the condition is not corrected fairly soon after birth, the heart becomes damaged beyond repair—the right ventricle is chronically overstrained driving blood through the arterial system, while the left is burdening the lungs with excessive pressures. Patients drag on in a state of chronic heart failure until they are transplanted or die.

Jan Quaegebeur, chief of the Columbia-Presbyterian congenital and pediatric cardiac practice, as much as anyone, brought the arterial switch into wide application. Smith describes him as a "colossus, the greatest congenital surgeon in the universe." Quaegebeur didn't invent the switch, Smith says, but "Jan was the first to publish a large series of switches with breathtakingly low mortality and was the most talented early adopter by far. Without someone like Jan to show that the concept could be translated into reproducible safe practice, it wasn't worth much."

Quaegebeur, "Q" to most of the staff, is Belgian, but spent the first twenty-plus years of his career at Leiden University in the Netherlands, with visiting-professor stints at both Harvard and Baylor, before being recruited to Columbia in 1990. Now sixty, he is a small, neat, soft-spoken man, who, at the mere whiff of a fool, transforms into a study in red-faced irritation. His speed and technical skills are legendary. Speed is not always a good sign in surgery, but Quaegebeur achieves it while looking unhurried: the procedure just flows by without wasted motion or a false step. (Argenziano points out that, step for step, Quaegebeur works at about the same speed as the other surgeons, but uses less time between steps. Since a complex operation might involve thousands of discrete steps, a few seconds' pickup at each one can create a striking time differential.)

The patient in the switch operation was a baby only five days old. Although she had been born somewhat prematurely, she looked plump and pink, almost an adman's ideal of the bouncing baby girl. But a sharp-eyed pediatrician had picked up subtle sonogram abnormalities during the pregnancy and ordered the tests that confirmed what terrible trouble this baby was in. Her great vessels were transposed, there were large holes in both her atrial and ventricular walls (hence the deceptive pinkness), her aortic arch was underdeveloped and rigid, and just beyond the arch the aorta had a deep dent, or "coarctation," simultaneously starving her lower body of oxygen while diverting too much pressure to the brain. Hardly a decade ago, she wouldn't have had a chance of surviving.

The operation was exhilirating. Over four-plus hours, Quaegebeur basically built the baby a new heart. He quickly opened the chest—babies' bones pose little resistance—laid a network of sutures to clear working space, and within just a few minutes had the baby on bypass. The basic steps sound straightforward: Quaegebeur first dissected and repaired the aortic arch and the coarctation by cutting out the diseased areas and splicing the healthy sections—unless the diseased areas are unusually large, the aorta will rebuild itself into a normal formation. He then dissected the pulmonary artery, removed the coronary arteries—which were misconnected to the pulmonary artery—and grafted them to their proper places on the new aorta. Since the baby's coronary arteries weren't much thicker than dental floss, he kept a button of flesh at each connection point to facilitate the suturing. Then he reconnected both the pulmonary artery and the new aorta to their proper locations. He used specially treated pieces of cadaver pericardium first to patch the openings where he had removed the coronary arteries and then to patch and repair the holes inside the baby's heart. (The pericardium acts as a natural scaffold to support new growth in the heart's interior walls; the treating process ensures both that it is sterile and won't generate a rejection reaction.) At about the three-and-a-half-hour mark, he closed the heart, warmed it, went off bypass, and spent long, careful minutes watching the echo image of its performance before nodding yes, it looked fine.

That summary obscures the dozens of crucial judgments Quaegebeur was making throughout the operation. The details of almost every step—where he cannulated for the bypass, how he dissected the two great arteries, where he reconnected the coronaries, how he remodeled the inside of the heart—depended on aspects of the deformations that he could not see until the chest was open. The consequences of making those calls incorrectly could be devastating—placing the coronaries too high or too low

on the new aorta, for instance, could lead to early blockages or a host of other downstream failures.

I had become used to feats of surgical concentration,
but Quaegebeur's demeanor through the operation seemed
to me almost trancelike, to the point where he was mur-
muring instructions to the perfusionist, Jeremy Tamari,
who was desperately straining to hear. Most of the time,
Quaegebeur's body was almost perfectly still, with only
his hands moving. (Artur Rubinstein played the piano that
way.) It struck me too that when he was cutting out his
pericardium patches, he didn't measure them first,
although there are a variety of measuring tools for surgeons. Smith had done the same thing when he was fash-
ioning his bypass graft networks—he would glance at the
heart, cut out his artery and vein pipeline sections, and
when he stitched them together, they fit, just as Quaegebeur's patches did.

This was also the one operation in which I managed to
embarrass myself. As usual, I positioned myself at the
head of the table so I could see everything but otherwise
tried to be more or less invisible. But most of the surgeons
would take a minute here and there to explain a procedure to me, and I got into the habit of asking the occasional question. So at one point, I asked Quaegebeur a
question. He didn't react for a moment, then stopped,
shook his head as if to clear it, and looked up, half in puz-
zlement and half in shock—"Did somebody *say* something? Who said something? Was there a *question*?" As I
was contemplating crawling under the table, Jonathan
Chen, the razor-sharp junior surgeon, suppressing a grin
and, it seemed to me, waiting at least two extra beats,

finally bailed me out by answering the question. Quaegebeur disappeared back into his own space.

When it was over, and the team was readying the baby
for the ICU, Quaegebeur walked me through the details of
the procedure and I asked about the baby's prognosis.
"Oh," he shrugged matter-of-factly, "I think she'll be
fine." And in fact, that's almost certainly true. The outcome data from these operations—the first cases are ten-
plus years old—are simply spectacular. Survival rates
exceed 90 percent, and more than 80 percent appear to
be leading normal lives, medically, academically, and
socially. It's hard to imagine a more unambiguous good.

The Rest of the Team

Beyond the surgical team proper—the surgeon, the resident, and the physician's assistant—the important supporting players are the anesthesiologists, the perfusionists,
and the OR nurses.

Anesthesiologists. In the real world, when you get
stabbed in the heart, you die. The anesthesiologist's job is
to facilitate an intrinsically assaultive operation with minimum disruption in vital functions—respiration, circulation, blood gases, chemical balances, urine output. Or as
Shanewise put it, "We keep the patients alive."*

---

*Although the several anesthesiologists I got to know seemed really to
enjoy their work—and it is among the best-paid medical specialties—
they sometimes conveyed a rueful sense of inferiority vis-à-vis the surgeons. "The surgeon always gets the case of wine, even though we
may have been the one who saved the patient," one told me. Surgeons

In beating-heart surgery, for example, one of the key challenges is to maintain stable hemodynamic pressure throughout the operation. While heart-lung machine pressures may be only approximate, they are at least consistent. In Craig Smith's off-pump quintuple bypass, however, when he used a suction device to lift and twist the heart to get to the rear coronaries, he had to be very careful not to squeeze the arteries shut. Beyond that, the mere fact that he clamped five different working arteries in rapid succession could have triggered sudden pressure losses throughout the heart.

It is the anesthesiologist who keeps a metaphorical finger on the pulse of the patient throughout such procedures, using an array of monitors—including a flow-measuring device threaded directly into the heart—and deploying a vast armory of pharmaceuticals. Just putting a patient "to sleep" usually involves three different drugs—a soporific, a painkiller (usually fentanyl, an opioid about eighty times more powerful than morphine), and a paralytic (to forestall involuntary muscle jerks). The surgery itself may entail a dozen or so others—vasodilators to reduce blood pressure and vasopressins to increase it, drugs to slow clotting and to speed it back up again, drugs to protect clotting mechanisms while they are being disrupted, and so on and on. There is an immense and constantly evolving literature on the timing, dosages, and blending of medications at

---

allegedly tell anesthesiologist jokes, the way violinists tell violist jokes. My favorite was the description of anesthesiologists as "the half-asleep looking after the half-awake," but I heard it from an anesthesiologist, not a surgeon.

every operative stage. "Every operation is a kind of scientific experiment," Johanna Schwarzenberger told me.

I got a better appreciation of the surgeon-anesthesiologist interplay during a pediatric procedure, an especially elegant operation to fix an aortic coarctation in a three-year-old boy. The lead surgeon was Ralph Mosca—he is in his mid-forties and, along with Quaegebeur, one of the two senior pediatric surgeons. A New Yorker, he did his cardiothoracic residency at Columbia-Presbyterian, then spent eight years concentrating in pediatric surgery at the University of Michigan before returning to Columbia in 2000. Schwarzenberger was the anesthesiologist, while the resident was Yasutaka Hirata. Hirata is a fully qualified cardiac surgeon in Japan, but is taking an additional pediatric residency at Columbia-Presbyterian. (Japanese surgeons often take residencies in the United States and Europe, he told me. In Japan, the cardiothoracic surgeons tend to provide many of the preparatory and follow-up services that surgical assistants and cardiologists provide in this country. The volume of actual surgeries each surgeon can handle is therefore much lower. By training abroad, they can get much faster exposure to a wide range of cases.)*

Mosca quickly opened the little boy's chest and pointed

---

*The broader pre- and postoperative role of the Japanese surgeon, while it sounds highly desirable from the standpoint of continuity of care, is probably not in patients' best interest. There is a massive body of data showing a high correlation between heart surgery volumes and outcomes. The same operation can evolve so differently from one patient to the next that it takes a lot of cases before a surgeon can react confidently to each new confluence of events. According to Hirata, forward thinkers in Japan would prefer to move toward the Western model, but it would create an instant surplus of surgeons.

to a lobelike organ on one side. "Do you know what that is?" he asked me. It looked like a lung, but was a gaudy lipstick-pink color. "All the adult lungs you've seen are black and purple, right?" he said. "Well, this is what they look like when we get them."

Repairing the coarctation required severing the aorta on either side of the dent and then suturing it back together. To avoid the heart-lung machine, they decided to clamp the aorta with a large L-shaped device that shut off blood flow below the coarctation as well as into two important arteries above, including the left carotid artery to the brain. While the right carotid could fully supply the brain during clamp time, the lower extremities would have to get by on circulation from collateral vessels, which they calculated would be safe for up to twenty minutes or so. Schwarzenberger attached a network of pressure monitors at multiple points on the child's body, and she and the surgeons agreed on their pressure objectives and modes of intervention. Their reference pressure scale was a systolic/diastolic average: the target was cranial pressure at the preclamp 72, and a minimum of 15 at the lower extremities.

When all the prep work was finished, Mosca applied the clamp and Hirata executed the operation. It took about three minutes to dissect and clean out the coarctation and to start the suturing. At one point, Mosca said quietly to Hirata, "I want you to go quickly, but don't rush. You'll get jerky." Hirata nodded and noticeably smoothed out his suturing. Schwarzenberger advised them on the time and the pressure readings on a minute-by-minute basis, and intervened with a drug infusion once when a lower extremity reading fell toward 16. Cranial pressures were steady at 72 throughout. At the sixteenth minute, as soon as the suturing was plausibly complete, Mosca unclamped. Lower extremity pressure jumped back into the 30s, and Schwarzenberger began coaxing it higher while Hirata and Mosca checked the sutures. There was one small leak, which Mosca closed off with a deft stitch or two, and they spent another five minutes cleaning up. By the time they finished, all the pressure monitors were reading an identical 72. Perfect. Total elapsed time was just over two hours—altogether a lovely piece of work by a top-flight team.

While Hirata was closing the chest, Mosca took me on a quick tour of the pediatric cardiac ICU and its collection of amazingly tiny babies. When we returned, the team was removing the drainage tube in the little boy's chest before taking him up to the ICU. "You're extubating already?" I said—I'd just been to a meeting about keeping postoperative chest tubes in for at least twenty-four hours. "That's with adults," Mosca said. "We can usually take it out right away. That's one of the reasons I like working on kids. They have better protoplasm."

The most difficult anesthesiology challenge, according to Sanford Littwin, another of the cardiothoracic anesthesiologists, is the off-pump double-lung transplant. The division does about fifty lung transplants a year and prefers to do almost all of them off-pump. For a single-lung transplant, with even a barely adequate second lung, keeping the patient oxygenated is fairly straightforward, Littwin says. But when the patient is already dying on two lungs, he can fall off the cliff when one of them is removed. Keeping him alive entails walking a physiologic tightwire—forcing oxygen volume through the remaining lung without rupturing anything, while administering heroic pharmaceutical infusions to widen the airpaths. And when something goes wrong, Littwin says, "there's no place in the notes where the anesthesiologist can hide. The surgeon can always say that a patient was 'anatomically unsuitable' for the operation, but when we screw up, it's really obvious."

Perfusionists. We've already seen the delicate pas de deux between Smith and Allison Cohen, the perfusionist in Mr. Goldfarb's valve replacement. Given the condition of his valve, a false step in easing him onto bypass could have seriously damaged his heart. The perfusionists at Columbia-Presbyterian are an exceptionally attractive group of young men and women, mostly in their early and mid-thirties, bright, articulate, and very knowledgeable about heart surgery. (Since I was spending so much time in the OR, I needed a convenient base between procedures, and made my quarters with them.) They are all college graduates, mostly science majors, who have completed one or two years of certification training, plus several years of on-the-job apprenticeship. They are well paid: starting salaries are in the $75,000 range, and experienced perfusionists command incomes well into the six figures.

Linda Mongero, the high-energy director of the unit, has been a perfusionist for twenty-seven years, most of them with Columbia-Presbyterian. Although her responsibilities are primarily managerial, she still does about eighty cases a year "to keep my hand in." "For two hours or so," Mongero says, "I am the patient's heart and lungs. The patient's life, quite literally, hangs on how well I do my job." The main challenge is to bring the patient on and off the machine with minimum disruption to blood pressure and circulation—a dramatic circulatory interruption or too-rapid surge from the bypass machine could throw a patient into lethal shock. But they also have an important piece of the monitoring assignment. Just moving the operating table up and down in the course of a surgery can cause blood-pressure changes. And the machine itself can be a source of problems—the filters can become clotted, for instance, possibly requiring a "bypass within the bypass machine." "You have to anticipate trouble," Mongero says. "Everybody's very tense during the surgery, but if we keep it smooth—just 'I'm changing a filter now . . . change complete'—there's no disruption." In keeping with the division's research imperative, Mongero and Jimmy Beck, the unit's assistant director, are working on a perfusion textbook, and Mongero is a coauthor with Smith on several peer-reviewed papers on hemodynamic management during surgery.

OR Nurses. The last set of major players in the OR are the nurses, and in the cardiothoracic division, the nursing staff, to a remarkable degree, is an extension of Flora Wang. Wang, a plump, cheerful, forceful woman—whom I first took to be about fifty—has been a nurse for forty-five years, and the senior cardiothoracic nurse for thirty-five. She trained in Taiwan and by the late 1960s had become the head OR nurse in Taiwan's newest medical center. Handpicked to nurse both Generalissimo and Madame Chiang Kai-shek during their surgeries, she impressed George Humphrey, then chairman of Columbia's surgery department, who was a consultant on the Chiangs' operations. Since she was interested in learning American cardiac methods, Humphrey recruited her to Columbia in 1971, initially just for a two-year rotation, which gradually became permanent. She naturally was in the OR during the Clinton surgery, so "I have operated on two heads of state," she laughs delightedly, pointing out that she also did Columbia's first heart transplant, first lung transplant, first liver transplant, and first LVAD (a near-equivalent to an artificial heart implant).

Although OR nurses were once trained by rotating them through all the surgical specialties, climaxing with open-heart, Wang now gets nurses fresh from school. She first assigns them to a several-week observation rotation to see if they can handle it: Is it too stressful? Can they handle the equipment? If they want to proceed, there is a second three-month observational-training regimen. If they still want to commit after that, she says, "then I *really* train them." It takes almost a year before they are at the table by themselves.

In heart surgery, Wang says, "Everything is speed. You have to move very fast. I tell them, 'Even when you set up the table in the morning, you have to rush.' They say, 'Why? There is plenty of time.' I say, 'The patient is there smiling, everything is fine, the anesthesiologist puts in a tube, and the patient arrests! The surgeon is calling for a knife, and you have to be ready! You set the table up fast, and if nothing happens, *then* you can relax until the surgery starts.'"

She goes on: "I tell them you have to know what the

surgeon wants, not what he *says* he wants, but what he really wants. Maybe he says he wants a scissors. But you're looking! You see the patient is bleeding! So why does he want a scissors? He means the clamp! You hand him the clamp!" And, she stresses, you have to work through mistakes. "You make a mistake," she says, "you *swallow* your mistake! There is no time to panic."

It would be hard to overestimate Wang's influence. She has, of course, trained all the cardiothoracic OR nurses, but she also takes new residents under her wing as well—and all the Columbia-Presbyterian cardiac attendings, except for Quaegebeur, started out as residents under Wang's watchful eye. When new residents make mistakes, she says, "They think it's so awful. I say, 'No! It happened! It's over! You *swallow* it! You stay calm. You keep working!' " She giggles: "They call me 'Momma.' "

There are practical aspects to Wang's suzerainty. For one thing, she keeps a gimlet eye on costs. Perfusionists are not allowed to open the sterile tubing while standing by during an off-pump operation. (Most of a bypass machine's tubing is reusable, but not the part that crosses the sterile field.) Going from off-pump to on-pump has to be fast, she says, "but the surgeon can't be ready in an instant. There's plenty of time to open the tubing. Otherwise, you're throwing away two thousand dollars! It's the same with sutures. Open what you need. Each one costs thirty dollars! Ten dollars! Five dollars!"

I had noticed how simple the cardiothoracic surgical-equipment tables were, and how they seemed identical for all the surgeons. Surgeons love gadgets. They all have favorite toys, and the instrument companies indulge them with dozens of models of the most basic instruments, like needle holders. When I asked Wang about it, she beamed. "We have a very limited equipment table," she said. "Nurses visit from other hospitals and complain that every one of their tables is different. I try not to allow the surgeons to use a different way. We work in this hospital, we use the same instruments, laid out the same way. Otherwise, you just make the nurse confused. Sutures the same thing, needleholders the same way. I want everybody to use the same set, same way. More instruments means more computers, more counts." The safety benefits from a uniform instrument table are obvious, but it's exactly the kind of issue that surgeons hate to take on, so controls can usually be imposed only by a strong external authority. Kudos to Flora Wang.

It's hard to overstate the importance of the artisanal, or artistic, skills in executing procedures like the ones I've been describing. But infrastructure and processes really matter as well—as is demonstrated by the current practice of transplant medicine.

Chapter 4

THE MOST PRECIOUS RESOURCE

ROGER ALTMAN IS CHAIRMAN AND FOUNDER OF one of the hotter boutique international investment banks, Evercore Partners, a firm that epitomizes a new mean-and-lean ethic on Wall Street. Although the firm has only about sixty professionals, a public offering in mid-2006 valued it at almost $600 million. Altman himself has drawn considerable attention for personally mediating the 2005 AT&T-SBC merger, one of the biggest of recent deals, and has been a key figure in the restructuring of General Motors. For several years in the late 1980s, I was a consultant to a bank where Roger was a senior partner, and worked on several transactions with him. He is Central Casting's prototype for the Wall Street mover-and-shaker—quick-moving and quick-thinking, a natural athlete, a horse and cattle rancher, an avid runner. So I was shocked when a mutual friend, who knew I was writing about heart surgeons, told me that Roger had had a heart transplant. By chance, I bumped into him a few weeks later at a policy forum we both belong to. I hadn't seen him for years, but he looked much the same, full of nervous energy, intense on his cell phone and BlackBerry. But, yes, he confirmed, he had indeed had a heart transplant, and we made an appointment to talk about it.

Altman discovered he had a heart problem in 1992 when he collapsed during a run in Central Park. The problem was "tachycardia" of the right ventricle: his heart would suddenly speed up to the point where the ventricle couldn't fill with blood. Over time, the episodes of rapid beats degenerated into fibrillations, or aimless flutters. The first line of defense was an implanted defibrillator, an electrical device that shocks the heart back into a normal rhythm. That worked to a point, but as the episodes weakened Altman's heart muscle, his ventricular walls thickened and stiffened, steadily losing their capacity to pump blood. By late 2001, a transplant was the only option. He was put on a waiting list, and checked into New York–Cornell medical center in the hope of staying alive until he got a match. After a two-month wait, his name came up, and he was transferred to Columbia-Presbyterian; Mehmet Oz did the surgery.

Within six months, Altman says, he was back to his normal life. That's a fast recovery, but one imagines that he was an extraordinarily determined patient. And the "normal life" of a transplant patient is not quite like anyone else's. "It's always in the front of your mind," he said. "For one thing, you're always walking the line between taking enough immune suppressant to prevent organ rejection, but not so much that you'll get pneumonia."

Opportunistic infections are a constant worry. "So far, I've been lucky," he said, but he avoids crowds, washes his hands frequently, and makes a wide berth around other people's illnesses. And his recovery has not been without complications. He had a serious kidney episode—probably from the anti-immune medication—but a different drug seems to have alleviated the problem. More recently, he has been worried by coronary artery blockages, which can be especially quick-developing in transplanted hearts. One blockage has been opened with a stent, and the doctors are tracking the other arteries carefully.

Altman, of course, knows all the numbers. The average transplant patient survives about twelve years, and at the time we talked, he was in the middle of his fifth. He still keeps himself in much better physical shape than most transplant recipients, and an average twelve-year survival rate, after all, means that half of the recipients survive longer, some much longer. Still, he spoke of the nearly five years since the transplant as a gift of extra time. Our conversation was by phone, a few days before the Labor Day weekend. Altman had left New York and was calling from his ranch. So while life was not perfect, it clearly beat the alternative.

OVER THE past five years, Columbia-Presbyterian has performed an average of nearly two heart transplants a week. That's about five times the volume at the next-busiest New York center, and far more than any other in the country. Since the number of U.S. heart transplants has been slowly dropping, Columbia-Presbyterian's share of the transplant business is steadily going up. Increased concentration in a specialty like transplants makes perfect sense. Good surgery goes with high volumes, and transplants require deep and experienced support teams that low-volume centers can't afford. Columbia-Presbyterian's one-year heart transplant survival rate has been running at about 95 percent, significantly above the 87–88 percent rate in the rest of the country.

To understand the process from start to finish, I decided to begin at the beginning.

Harvest Run

I got the call about 9:30 on a Friday night, from Joe Costa, Craig Smith's physician's assistant, who does double duty a couple of weeks a month as an organ-collection team leader. "I think we have one," he said. "We're not taking the heart, it looks like, but we will take a lung." (The division's lung surgeons do about a third as many transplants as the cardiac section, but that still accounts for almost all lung transplants in the state.) He told me to meet him in front of the hospital at midnight. Costa has been a physician's and surgeon's assistant for eight years and is board-certified in both internal medicine and surgery. He has the no-nonsense, can-do bearing of an army master sergeant and, with hundreds of harvests under his belt, is one of the most experienced organ-collection hands in the hospital.

Columbia-Presbyterian is in northern Manhattan near the George Washington Bridge. When I got there, Costa explained that the donor was at a small hospital in west-

ern New York. A hospital van would take us to Teterboro
Airport in New Jersey, where we would catch an executive
jet service to an airport near the donor hospital. He
didn't know who the other teams would be, he said, but
he hoped they were experienced.

Other teams? It hadn't occurred to me, but a good
organ donor would naturally have more than just a heart
or a lung on offer. There were typically four teams at a
harvest, Costa said—heart, lung, liver, and kidney/
pancreas—so there was a natural division between "belly
guys" and "chest guys." Since the belly and chest teams
were shoulder-to-shoulder, working space could get con-
tentious. "I was just on a run where an older surgeon
working on the liver was really using his elbows," he said,
"until I confronted him and told him to stop. Then, supposedly by accident, he let an intestine flop into the chest
area. It was really irritating. If you have good teams,
everyone knows the rules and you help each other." I had
a momentary flash of panic—a Grand Guignol vision of a
dim basement morgue where men with long knives plun-
dered a bloody corpse. I decided to keep it to myself.

It was about 12:30 A.M. when we left the hospital.
Besides Costa, the team included Mark Russo, a crisp and
confident young man taking a break from a nearly finished Columbia surgical residency to work in the cardiothoracic research labs, and Mike Glithero, a lab assistant
who was picking up overtime by lugging the organ transport gear, a big, picnic-style ice chest on wheels. Two affa-
ble executive jet pilots met us at the airport and ushered
us out to the waiting Lear. They turned out to be harvest-
run regulars, greeting Costa and Russo by name. "Is it

another lung?" one of them asked, and hoped our luck was changing. Five consecutive lung runs, I had learned in the van, had turned up unusable organs, as if through some malign intervention by the transplant gods. Each failed harvest is a huge letdown—by the time a "no-organ" report comes in, the surgical team is assembled, the hopeful recipient is usually already being prepped in the OR, and his family is at the hospital.

We arrived upstate about 1:30, and a hospital ambulance met us to take us to the donor site. Craig Smith had cautioned me a few weeks before about the atmospherics of a harvest. "Every donor represents a tragedy," he said. "And the better the donor, the worse it is. The groom's brother has too much to drink and falls off a balcony—you constantly see things like that." He warned me to be especially guarded if the harvest site was at a small hospital. "There may be only one entrance," he said, "and families sometimes hang around even after all the papers have been signed. So you may be parading by them in the waiting room. They'll know you're the harvest team, so you can't be talking or laughing."

It was a relief when we pulled up to a basement entrance—no gauntlet of family members—and by that time, I'd figured out that the harvest would be much like a regular surgery. You can't recover a heart or a lung from a corpse. While the donors must have been certified as brain-dead, they also must be on life support, so vital functions are more or less intact. And you would have no hope of preserving the harvested organ unless the "explant," or extraction, followed the same obsessively sterile protocols as any other open operation.

A nurse met us at the entrance, directed us back to the OR, and showed us where to get surgical caps and masks. A liver team from the Mount Sinai Medical Center in New York had already arrived, along with a kidney surgeon from a nearby regional medical school. The hospital had supplied an anesthesiologist, a surgical resident, and a young, cheerful scrub nurse. The donor was a man in his early fifties, with remarkably pink, young-looking skin. When we came into the OR, the locals and the Sinai team were well into creating the sterile field and draping the body. The only difference from a normal operation was the burly aide off to one side of the room at a table covered with bags of ice. He was wrapping each bag in the ubiquitous OR blue towels and methodically crushing the ice with a mallet.

The basic harvest procedure starts much as any other surgery, except that you're opening both the chest and the abdomen. The heart and liver teams usually do the openings, secure the working space, and then place sutures so their organs can be tied off as they're removed. As they finish, the lung and kidney teams take over the table to prepare their organs. The initial preparation takes about an hour and a half. When everything's ready, the heart team empties the heart into the chest by cutting a rear heart vein and the vena cava, the big trunkline bringing blood back to the heart, and injects protective cardioplegia. Both the belly and chest teams cross-clamp the aorta. The whole body cavity is dumped full of ice and allowed to cool for a few minutes. After the ice is vacuumed out, the heart team severs the pulmonary veins, the aorta and the pulmonary artery, lifts out the heart, flushes it further with cardioplegia to prevent spontaneous beating, then places it into a plastic ice bag that is buried in the ice in the organ carrier. The liver comes out just after the heart, and the lungs and kidneys follow in their turn, each being treated with roughly similar flushing and rinsing routines.

Cross-clamping the aorta triggers the countdown of the critical out-of-body period—the so-called cold ischemic time, or CIT. For an adult heart, survival rates are roughly unaffected within CITs of 250 minutes or so, but there is a marked survival falloff after about 300 minutes. For comparison, if we had been taking this donor's heart back to Columbia-Presbyterian, the total elapsed time before the heart was restarted would have been in the 150-to-200-minute range. Time tolerances for other organs are generally more forgiving. In a pinch, kidneys can even be taken from cadavers within the first day or so after cardiac death, with only somewhat degraded results.

As the explant got under way about 2:15, it dawned on me what hard duty this was for the workers at the donor hospital. An OR in a hospital of this size rarely does a chest opening, and now strangers had appeared in the middle of the night and were demanding instruments and other facilities that they didn't have or couldn't find. The nurse was especially beleaguered—working by herself, instead as part of a two-nurse team, and servicing two surgical teams for procedures she'd never seen before—but she stayed upbeat and generally managed to keep pace. It was one of many heartening instances researching this book when I saw quite modestly paid people working very hard under great pressure—because it was the right thing to do.

The kidney surgeon generously put himself at the end of the organ queue and more or less took over the role of circulating nurse. He'd obviously done rounds at the hospital and knew where the odd piece of gear was stored, several times leaving the OR to dig it up himself. The sternal saw, for opening the chest, wouldn't start, so Costa finally asked for a "blade." I think only the kidney surgeon knew what he meant, but he went out and returned with a tool from preelectric-saw days—a long, sturdy, stainless steel knife accompanied by a large steel mallet. Costa positioned the blade, hooking it under the sternum and holding it upright, and told the surgical resident to drive it with the mallet. "No, *pound* it!" he said after a couple of tentative pokes, and amid much clanging, the sternum was sliced smoothly through.

Costa and Russo had met members of the Sinai team before, and they worked well together, conveying instruments back and forth like a bucket brigade. I had never seen an abdominal opening, and was again surprised how little blood there was. All of the organs stood out in strikingly different colors, much as in plastic high school biology models. And I was fascinated to see the Sinai leader carefully gather the intestines and assemble them into a basketball-sized sphere completely wrapped in blue towels. When he finished, the abdominal cavity was almost completely clear—no flopping intestines—and he could easily move the blue basketball whenever it was in the way.

While Costa worked on the chest, Russo and the anesthesiologist were taking bronchoscopic readings on the lungs and running other tests. The donor had died from a cerebral event—more than that wasn't clear—and the heart had shown symptoms of chronic failure. Chronic heart and lung failure often go hand in hand; it was already clear that one lung was unacceptable, and the second one was looking doubtful. About 3:30, when it was just about time to ice down the body, Russo ran one more test, rapidly inflating the "good" lung to see how fast it deflated. A healthy lung deflates like a balloon when the plug is removed. This one took more than a minute, evidence of major obstructions. Another failed lung run.

We packed up quickly and left just as the belly team was putting in their ice. The good news was that both the liver and the kidneys looked like healthy organs. Bad heart and lungs notwithstanding, this donor's act of grace, in all likelihood, would save three lives.

When we got back to the airport, the pilots seemed as upset as Costa and Russo—six bad lungs may have been some kind of a record. On the way home, I heard Russo making a follow-up call to Josh Sonett—since appointed head of the thoracic section. "Yes, Josh," Russo was saying, "but believe me, you would *not* have given anyone that lung. . . ." It had been several weeks since the unit had made a lung transplant, an unusually long hiatus, there was a long waiting list, and tensions perhaps were beginning to show. It was Sunday morning, about 5:30, and the four of us were tired and a bit glum as we rolled into the Columbia-Presbyterian driveway. Costa and Russo were checking their messages. "Hey, we may have another lung," Russo said. "This one's local. Could be about ten A.M." All at once, they looked fresh and enthusiastic again.

Playing God

When we made the harvest run, I had only a rudimentary notion of how organs are matched with patients, but it was clear some higher-level system was involved. Russo got a call from "the OPO" checking on our progress on the trip out, and called them back on the way home to report the failed organ recovery. OPO, he told me, stood for "organ procurement organization." The matching system, in fact, as I learned over the next few weeks, is an unusually elegant example of cooperative public-private, national-local problem-solving.

The first successful human organ transplants date from the late 1950s (kidneys) and late 1960s (hearts), and by the 1980s, transplant technology was entering the medical mainstream. Craig Smith's first postresidency assignment at Columbia-Presbyterian in 1984 was to create their heart-lung transplant program. Today, annual U.S. transplant volumes run at about 13,000 kidneys (about half of them donated by living relatives), 6,500 livers, 2,100 hearts, and 1,100 lungs, all with very high survival rates. Probably 200,000 Americans are walking around with a functioning organ from someone else's body.

The overall matching system is supervised by a private nonprofit agency established by Congress in 1984. The enabling legislation was substantially revised in 1998 with the aim of improving fairness and reducing disparities in outcomes. "Medical urgency" is still a major selection criterion, but mere closeness to death isn't an automatic qualifier, since matchings must "avoid wasting organs [or making] . . . futile transplants." Rigid allocation rules, such as residence or length of time on the list, are specifically disallowed. In principle, the highest-ranking candidate for an organ could be anywhere in the country; in practice, especially for hearts, which are the most perishable, a qualified recipient will have to be within the zone imposed by cold ischemic time limitations.

The detailed matching is done through a national computer system that uses a formula to match waiting-list patients with available organs in rank order of suitability. The foot soldiers of the matching process, however, are the local OPOs, each one serving an area of about 9 million people. The New York City OPO, covering the 110 hospitals within the metropolitan area, is run by Eric Grossman, a Harvard-trained nephrologist. As Grossman explained it, all hospitals are required by law to make a telephone report to the local OPO on every actual or impending death. In New York, that translates into about 55,000 calls a year. An initial filter—primarily whether the patient is on life support—narrows those down to about 1,800 potential donors. A telephone screening for infections, major cancers, or similar conditions eliminates about another third. Everyone else gets an on-site visit by a transplant-trained nurse, usually within two hours of the initial call. For a potential heart donor, the nurse documents any previous heart trouble, and retrieves, or orders, an echocardiogram. If a patient is a good prospect, but the family hasn't made a decision to donate, a donation counselor will visit to secure their approval. Ideally, Grossman says, the legal processes can be completed before the patient is certified as brain-dead, so there will be minimum loss of time between the certification (by two separate neurologists) and the activation of a harvest.

If the legal requirements are in place, and the computer has turned up potential recipients, the OPO nurse at the donor hospital calls the transplant centers in order of recipient rank, to determine whether the patient is available and in transplantable physical condition. The center almost always asks for additional tests—a new echo, blood gases, the heart's responsiveness to stimulants. There are time limits on the decision-making. "We try not to be too rigid," Grossman said, "but sometimes you get the feeling that they're on the fence or that you're talking to a resident who's asking for more tests because he's waiting for his attending to wake up. Then you just have to say, "Okay, are you taking the heart, or are you not taking the heart?'".

While the match is made by a computer, the decision whether someone actually gets *on* a list, and his medical urgency classification, is made by local transplant committees. At Columbia-Presbyterian, the adult transplant coordinating committee meets every Friday morning, chaired jointly by Yoshifumi Naka, the transplant surgery program director and Donna Mancini, a professor of medicine and director of the Center for Advanced Cardiac Care, who oversees transplant cardiology. There are usually about thirty people around the table—transplant cardiologists, social workers, psychiatrists, infection specialists, neurologists, surgeons, transplant nurses, and others. Most of the cardiologists are from Mancini's section, but very occasionally an outside cardiologist may attend as well, to help advocate a listing for one of his patients.

Committee meetings open with a review of the current

IF YOU WANT
TO BE A DONOR

Simply checking a box on your driver's license is not likely to result in an organ donation. Even if you fill out a formal donor's card, few hospitals will take an organ over family objections. To be sure that you will be considered as a donor, take the following steps:

1. Complete the state organ and tissue donor registration form. Almost every state maintains a registry, and the forms are usually available from state Web sites.
2. Stipulate in your will and other legal directives that you wish to be a donor. Designate an individual who understands your wish to donate and grant him or her the authority to sign the required documentation.
3. TELL YOUR CHILDREN AND SPOUSE about your intention. The hospital may also ask them to sign the authorizing documents.

All major religions have endorsed organ and tissue donations. Many people also report that the thought of a loved one living on through the gift of life to others eases the pain of bereavement.

There are few age limitations on donating; even very old people can become donors.

waiting list, followed by an intense case review of recent transplants. Few patients are ever the focus of so much concentrated medical brainpower. Transplant X has an intestinal infection: is that resolving itself or are we overdoing the immunosuppressants? Transplant Y is refusing to get out of bed: is she depressed? The psychiatrists will follow up. Here are Transplant Z's blood chemistries, and last week's trends: what does the group think? The lavishness of the resources partly reflects the value of the sunk investment. It's not just money—although at $200,000 to $300,000 per patient, transplants are stunningly expensive. The "most precious resource of all," in Naka's words, is the donated heart, which is quite literally priceless. An early death of a transplant patient is therefore uniquely tragic— not only has a patient died, but a rare gift has been wasted, a donor's good intentions flouted, and another patient who might have been more suitable may now die as well.

Finally, the meeting focuses on new candidates for listing—there were two or three at each of the meetings. The twin questions were: Should this person be listed for a transplant? And what urgency level should she be assigned?* The medical criteria seemed the easiest to apply. People are disqualified for transplants if they're

---

*In 1999, two urgency statuses, 1 and 2, were refined to 1A, 1B, and 2. 1Bs from the donor region, which involves several OPOs, will get priority over a 1A from an outside region, in part because of cold ischemic time limitations. The 2 status is becoming controversial. As cardiology improves, waiting-list death rates are dropping, and some 2s have been on the list for years, some for more than ten years. When the survival rate on the list exceeds that of a successful transplant, Naka points out, that person prima facie shouldn't be listed—"A transplant is a dangerous operation."

"too sick or too well," in Naka's words. The "too sick" hurdle is quite a high one—a presentation at one committee involved a patient with both heart failure and renal failure. He had received his new heart the previous night and was scheduled for a new kidney that afternoon. He was doing fine.

The hardest discussions involved a candidate's psychosocial status. Put baldly, the question was: can this patient be trusted with a new heart? Substance abusers—drug addicts, alcoholics, smokers—were automatically out. Obesity was another disqualifier, although the threshold is high—a person five and a half feet tall would have to weigh over 216 pounds to be denied listing. Getting off the drugs or losing weight, however, could move a patient onto the list, but the committee had to be convinced that the patient would stick with it. (I sat in on a review, at another committee, of a lung transplant case involving a former polysubstance abuser. He had suffered an overdose of fentanyl, the powerful opioid used in surgery. The hospital had dosed him correctly, but his parents were smuggling in "fentanyl lollipops."* And then there was the heart transplant patient caught hiding bags of Cheetos in his intensive care bed.)

Discussions focused hard on evidence of personal discipline. In one case, a cardiologist blurted out in exasperation about a candidate, "He has lousy teeth. He won't go to the dentist!" He was not listed. Not having health insurance is usually disqualifying. "It's not that the hospi-

---

*No joke. Fentanyl is sometimes supplied in berry-flavored lozenges, prescribed especially for patients with advanced cancers. There is inevitably an active street market.

tal won't get paid for the surgery," Naka said, "but a patient without insurance won't maintain his medications or his follow-up program." (I believed him on the payment question: Columbia-Presbyterian performs a lot of uninsured surgery, and an outside cardiologist told me he'd sent them seven Medicaid transplant patients within the past two years, all guaranteed money-losers.)

There is an uncomfortable edge of class bias in those decision criteria, even though surgeons tell you that they don't make moral judgments on their patients. Mehmet Oz told me a story from his days as a Columbia surgical resident. He was a superb ER surgeon, and so naturally fell into the triage role. This was the high-crime "Fort Apache" era in New York City, when ERs were overwhelmed, and it was up to Oz to decide who got cared for and in what order. One night the police brought in three shooting victims. "There was a dead cop," Oz said. "Next to him was the shooter, who was in critical condition, and then there was a pregnant woman who was caught in the cross fire. She was badly hurt but stable. I saw the three of them and realized that I wanted the shooter to die. At the same time, the staff are looking at me to decide—this all took seconds. And I pointed at the shooter. He's next. We can't help the cop, and the woman's stable, so we save the shooter. The next day," Oz went on, "the police discovered that the *woman* was the shooter—she was running a drug den—and the man was just some guy walking by. That case had a profound effect on me. We can't make judgments about who deserves to live."

I gradually understood, however, that no surgeon would see a contradiction between Oz's parable and the ranking of transplant candidates. The surgical worldview is, has to be, insistently factual, but within the fact-set defined by the profession. Saddam Hussein and Mother Theresa both arrive at the ER. They can both be saved if the surgeon does Hussein first, but Hussein will die if Mother Theresa goes first. It's a no-brainer—Hussein will always go first. The same logic dictates the selection for transplants. Person A will take care of a new heart and so, odds are, will live longer. Person B is not likely to take care of it, and odds are, will die sooner. Person A gets it. That may not be fair. But the transplant is about the *heart*, and getting a maximum life span out of that very precious heart.

If anyone objected to those decision criteria, I saw no sign of it. Committee discussions were often intense—about *whether* an individual would stay off cigarettes, for instance—but never about the principles involved. Nor did I ever see a vote. The discussion would proceed to a point. Someone would say, "Well, let's make her a 1B." Or, "I don't think he should be listed." Everyone would nod and the meeting would move on. It was the same mode of consensual decision-making that had so impressed me at the surgical meetings. I mentioned it once to Naka, and he just shrugged: "We have a long history."

Donna Mancini also happened to be Roger Altman's transplant cardiologist. He told me that, while he was grateful for Oz's execution of the surgery, "it's Donna who keeps me alive." Transplant cardiologists, Mancini explained, must take over the supervision of all their patients' care, for the transplant dominates all subsequent medical interactions. Even for a "normal" injury, like a broken leg, she said, "we have to be involved in the medication a patient gets. It's actually a wonderful practice—one of the few specialties where you're really involved with every aspect of patient care."

Naka readily concurred. The cardiologist, not the surgeon, is the true "transplant doctor," he said. A transplant center gets notified about a match only hours before the surgery happens, so the surgeon is whichever one is on the call rotation. (Mike Argenziano, Allan Stewart, and Naka handle all the adult heart transplants.) "In normal heart surgery," Naka said, "you know the patients. You've met with them and their families several times, know their histories, discussed alternatives. But when I'm called for a transplant, it's almost always the first time I've seen the patient." The surgeon obviously stays involved as necessary and checks on the patient in the ICU. But once the critical postsurgical days are past, he has little more to do.

Transplants, in fact, are considered one of the technically simplest of heart surgeries. Like most laymen, I found that surprising, but after I had seen one, it was clear why. In contrast to, say, working with coronary arteries and valves, a transplant involves only the largest anatomical structures, ones that are easy to see and easy to reach, and there is plenty of working space. Naka said that transplants are often the first procedure a new resident is allowed to do. "The attending can see every stitch, and if the resident makes a mistake, he can easily fix it."

I was the more struck, therefore, by the high degree of emotional content that transplants seem to hold for even the most seasoned surgeons. I think every surgeon I spoke to about transplants mentioned the eerie feeling of seeing the empty space in the chest after a heart has been removed. Eeriest of all, said Smith, was in the days of full heart-lung transplants, which are rare now, when the living patient was lying on the table with nothing at all in his thoracic cavity. And Smith's face flushed as he told me that the first moment after a transplant is finished and the heart fills with blood and starts to beat "is like watching a baby being born."

I will describe an actual transplant in the next chapter, but first I want to digress briefly to the emergence of a transplant alternative—the heart-assist device.

The Coming of the Mechanical Heart

"Destination" is a harsh word: it means this is it, the best we can do, the end of the road. The man on the operating table was a typical candidate for a "destination" assist device—mid-seventies, too old for a transplant, still thinking and speaking clearly, but so exhausted from chronic heart failure that he could do little but lie in bed. Dying ventricular muscle often swells and stiffens, and his chest images showed a heart almost the size of a soccer ball, one that, compared with a normal heart, could pump mere trickles of blood. This patient was never going to be "cured." But with a little luck, the assist device will keep him alive for a few more years at a considerably better functioning level than his present one.

Naka, the divisional assist-device guru, and Mauricio Garrido were the surgeons. This was in the fall of 2006. Garrido had completed his cardiothoracic residency, but had chosen to do an additional six-month fellowship in assist devices. Assist-device placements are often difficult operations, and this one promised to be particularly so. Like most destination candidates, this patient had undergone several heart surgeries, so there was a severe buildup of sticky scar tissue, which was all the more daunting because of the great size of the heart. Worried that the patient couldn't withstand the trauma of a long chest opening, they set up the bypass connections before they opened the chest—the aortal cannula was placed through an incision in the collarbone area, while the venous cannula was placed in the femoral, a big leg vein. If anything went wrong, they could get him on bypass within seconds.

Surgeons' fees for assist devices have only recently been raised to the level paid for transplants, although transplants are usually the easier operation, since there is no requirement to preserve the existing heart. Had this been a transplant operation, Naka and Garrido would have turned on the bypass machine right away and opened the chest without worrying about preserving the old heart. Instead, it took hours of patient, cautious scalpel work to get the chest open and the heart exposed. And before they could place the assist device, they also had to repair a grotesquely stretched mitral valve. Mitral repair is an expert's procedure—it is not only technically challenging, but requires considerable experience to recognize whether a valve is reparable and to choose the right approach. In this case, once they were on-pump, Naka and Garrido opened the heart to expose the valve, trimmed the valve leaflets, stitched in an artificial valve ring to pull the valve and the leaflets into a normal shape, and placed a ring of bracing stitches to prevent restretching.

The patient was getting an LVAD—a left ventricular assist device—which is the most common. The Thoratec HeartMate II assist device that Columbia-Presbyterian uses can be configured to support either ventricle, or both if necessary. Conceptually, its workings are simple. When the left ventricle fills with blood, it is drained away into an LVAD tube placed through the apex, or bottom point, of the heart. The LVAD motor drives the blood through another tube into the aorta just below the arch, with enough power for normal circulation—a left-ventricle mini bypass machine.

The surgery is conceptually just as simple. Sewing in the ventricular and aortal tubing is not much harder than placing bypass cannulae. Just as there is a "Columbia way" to place an aortic bypass cannula, Naka insists on an exact stitching pattern for the LVAD tubes, since they must withstand high pressures for years. In this case, however, before they could place the ventricular tube, Naka had to expose the apex. The heart was so big that, even with the sternal incision ratcheted as wide open as possible, the apex was hidden down underneath the chest. Inevitably, it was also stuck in some lingering scar tissue, which took more tedious, crouched-down scalpel work to remove. Then when the apex was freed, and Naka tried to pull it into the sternal opening, it kept slipping out of his hands—everything was slick with blood—and sliding back under the chest. I had a flash of a man I had once seen struggling to control a large halibut he had landed in a small boat.

When both LVAD tubes were finally in place, the surgeons carved out a pouch in the fatty area of the lower chest, inserted the LVAD, secured it with a couple of sutures, and ran a small external power line from the LVAD out through the chest wall. It took another twenty minutes or so to start up the LVAD, tune it to the right settings, and wean the patient off bypass. Everything seemed to work fine. All that was left was to clean up and close the chest.

Start to finish, the procedure took nearly eight hours. It occurred to me that it would be recorded in a dry couple-paragraph case report that would note the presence of cardiomegaly (the enlargement) and say that they had pre-positioned the bypass cannulae, opened the chest, removed adhesions, repaired the mitral valve—specifying the ring-type—and placed a Thoratec HeartMate II LVAD "in the usual manner." And that the operation had proceeded without incident. That would, indeed, be both true and complete, and somehow not begin to capture what had gone on.

State-of-the-art LVADs can pump the full range of a normal adult's requirements, even at full exercise, and will adjust their pumping rate to accord with oxygen consumption. The model that I had seen Naka and Garrido place is one of the newest—simpler, smaller, and less obtrusive than previous versions. The patient will wear two cell-phone–sized battery holsters, plus a somewhat larger control module, usually at the belt. At home, he will have a power module/battery recharger and a display console for readouts on his device status. The batteries provide about three hours of unconnected mobility; at home especially while resting or sleeping, he would normally connect to the power module.

On average, placing a destination LVAD costs about $200,000, or about the same as a transplant. The device itself costs $60,000 to $70,000, or probably at least as much as the all-in cost of an organ harvest. The median life expectancy of a patient on a destination device, however, is only about eighteen months. Those numbers were computed on older devices, and the newer models should do rather better, but that has yet to be proven. The total cost of the intervention, moreover, is far more than just that of the LVAD placement—extending the lives of very sick people will inevitably make large additional demands on the medical system.

So why do we do it? To begin with, this patient's procedure was part of a forty-plus-year effort by the federal government and major academic medical centers to develop an artificial heart. The first workable devices date from the 1960s; key names are the Texas Heart Institute's Denton Cooley and Baylor's Michael DeBakey, while Texas Instruments built the devices. (Frictions over precedence and control led to the bitter Cooley-DeBakey rivalry that seems to have eased only recently.) Another famous, or notorious, milestone was the "Jarvik heart," invented by Robert Jarvik and placed in sixty-one-year old Barney Clark at the University of Utah in 1982. Clark survived for 112 days, although his "life" was a horrifying sequence of catastrophic organ collapses and heroic interventions, interspersed by brief periods when Clark was awake and lucid. The total federal investment in artificial heart development by that point was $160 million.

In part because of widespread revulsion at the Clark episode, the research focus shifted to "bridge-to-transplantation" assist devices, primarily LVADs, rather than full-blown artificial hearts. By the mid-1990s, however, as the devices got smaller and more reliable, it became obvious that they could support at least some transplant-list patients for long periods of time. Eric Rose, Columbia's surgery department chairman, led a three-year twenty-two-center randomized trial of the LVAD as a destination device (the REMATCH* study) that reported in 2001. The study, which cost about $25 million, was funded by the federal government, Thoratec, and to a great extent, the participating universities. Half of the LVAD patients survived for a year, and a quarter made it to two years or longer. By comparison, only a quarter of the controls lived for a year, and only 8 percent for two years. The LVAD patients also enjoyed a much better quality of life, as measured by activity, mobility, and incidence of depression. As a consequence, the Thoratec device was approved by the FDA for general usage, and after lobbying by Rose and other of the trial's leaders, Medicare agreed to support destination assist devices, despite their price tag.

Two hundred thousand dollars for an additional year or so of life is still a lot of money—at some point we all have to die.† (To be fair, the REMATCH protocols specified that only patients with no other options could qualify, so they were an especially debilitated population. Malnutrition was an important factor in death rates.) What's interesting about the REMATCH study, however, as Annetine

---

*Randomized Evaluation of Mechanical Assistance for the Treatment of Congestive Heart Failure. Clinical trial managers have an apparently incurable weakness for clever acronyms.

† The cost of LVADs compares favorably with that of cancer drugs that are approved based on the basis of additional survival times of only weeks or months. Accumulating examples of high-cost, low-survival treatments doesn't justify them, of course.

Gelijns, the codirector of Columbia's InCHOIR,* points out, is that LVAD patient deaths were heavily tied to *device* problems, like device-related bleeding, placement-related infections and inflammation, and outright pump failure. And those are precisely the kinds of problems that technology is good at solving. Naka told me that, although the Thoratec device is improving, few of the component technologies are truly leading-edge. The gaiting factor, it seems, is not so much the nature of the challenge, but the size of the market. Total annual destination LVAD placements are probably still only in the hundreds. While big companies with deep investment capabilities are clearly interested, the market leaders are venture-style small companies with limited capital.

LVADs, in short, have the hallmarks of a technology on the cusp of a major breakout. One straw in the wind is the emergence of "continuous flow" devices. The REMATCH LVAD, like virtually all other assist devices to that point, was "pulsatile"—it used a diaphragm and pneumatic pressure to beat like a normal heart—and diaphragm problems were a major source of REMATCH failures. Recent development has focused on rotary pumps and constant flows. The new Thoratec model I saw implanted is such a device, and is much smaller and simpler than the one used in the REMATCH trials, which should result in fewer placement infections and longer service life.† (Once, as a guest on hospital cardiology

---

*International Center for Heart Outcomes and Innovation Research. (Cleverer than most, I admit.)
†Allan Stewart is involved in a research project on the physiological and chemical consequences of continuous-flow devices. Although it is

rounds, I heard a cardiologist explain continuous-flow devices to the residents. Several of his patients had them, but he said he still "freaked out a bit" when he placed a stethoscope and there was no heartbeat—just a steady *shhhhhhh*. Blood-pressure readings give a single number.) There is even an experimental continuous-flow device that is small enough to be placed directly into the heart via a catheter, without any surgery at all. Currently, it can give support for up to a week. Michael DeBakey, now in his mid-nineties, is a major force in the development of continuous-flow technology.

Another such straw is the freestanding destination assist-device center being developed at New York University Medical Center by Ulrich Jorde. Jorde is a transplant cardiologist whom I'd met when he was presenting one of his cases at a Columbia-Presbyterian committee meeting. He had trained and practiced at Columbia-Presbyterian before being recruited to NYU. The recruiters had contacted him, he said, because they wanted to build a transplant practice. "I asked them why they would do that, when the country's premier center is only six miles away." Instead, he convinced them that the opportunity is in LVADs. Because of their history as bridge-to-transplant devices, LVADs were only available in transplant centers.

---

at an early stage, it appears that the change to continuous flow causes some degree of organ shock. Interestingly, if a patient with a continuous-flow device gets a transplanted heart after several weeks on the device, there appears to be a *second* shock as the body adjusts back to pulsatile mode. That suggests that true bridge-to-transplant patients may be better off with pulsatile devices, while destination patients would use continuous-flow devices for longevity.

Jorde's program may be the world's first freestanding destination LVAD center. He's still building a team, but says he has had no trouble recruiting stars. NYU has done three LVADs so far and is cautiously looking to build volumes. He and Naka are friends, and he said the whole Columbia team has been very helpful. Like Naka, he also stressed the high hurdle posed by the current "device"—meaning the transplanted heart. "A transplanted heart now lasts on average for twelve years," Jorde said. "That's a tough standard." But he thinks that we're "just one step away" from a device that will be truly competitive.

Plausibly, within a decade or so, heart transplants will begin to give way to long-term assist devices. Two thousand transplants a year doesn't begin to meet current demand. Greater volume will drive down prices and speed the pace of improvement. As the cost of an assist device drops toward that of, say, a defibrillator, and the placement becomes safer and less invasive, patients will get them at an earlier stage of heart failure instead of waiting until they're near death. Healthier patients will improve survival performance. Patient numbers, equipment markets, and medical spending will all expand mightily.

The LVAD story is a parable for almost all of health care technology. The same cycles can be traced in CABGs, stents, cataract surgery, hip replacements, MRIs, and much else. Viewed solely through an economist's cost-benefit lens, a $200,000 LVAD placement looks like a misallocation of resources. Seen as a one-day snapshot near the end point of a half-century-long cycle, it tells rather a different story.

Chapter 5

ERIKA'S STORY

I SAW ERIKA MAYNARD ONLY ONCE. SHE WAS A heartbreakingly beautiful little girl of four, hugging a stuffed animal and in tears because her mother, Traci, had just stepped back so the nurses could take Erika into the OR to receive a new heart. This was the same little girl who was caught on a family video just the year before, all bright eyes and arc-light smile, shimmying in a lively dance. I was there to observe the transplant, and as the OR's double doors swung shut, I saw Traci shrink back against the corridor wall, with both hands over her mouth and terrible pain in her eyes.

The cases I've written about so far have mostly been accounts of amazing deeds and technical marvels. But Erika never woke up after her operation and died twelve days later. The entire kit of marvels mustered by cardiologists and surgeons in three states had not been up to the task of saving her.

Her story captures how a catastrophic illness like a failing heart consumes a family, and offers a glimpse at how Traci and her husband, Rich, are managing to knit their lives back together after Erika's death. But most of all, it is a corrective to the mirage of omnipotent medicine.

Getting to Columbia-Presbyterian

Muscatine sits on the hilly west bank of the Mississippi, across from Illinois, on the edge of Iowa corn country. Rich and Traci live in one of the town's lovely, leafy, residential enclaves hidden behind the crisscrossing interstates. I visited there late one Sunday morning in September 2006, about three months after Erika's death. Traci was still at church when I arrived—she helps out with children's programs—but Rich had come home to put their youngest, Evan, down for his nap. Their house, spacious and comfortably furnished, sits on a cul-de-sac with a large lawn, some mature trees, and a wooded hillside falling away from the back yard. While we were waiting for Traci, Rich showed me the garden, with a carved stone memorial to Erika that the two of them had begun constructing in the first agonizing weeks of their grief.

Traci arrived a half hour later with Emma, who had started first grade a few days before—Emma is pretty and athletic, but with unusual gravitas for a seven-year-old. Evan woke up shortly after, a bright, blond, gabbling, eighteen-month-old. Rich's mom, Mary, still slender and youthful-looking, showed up a while later to look after the kids. I had come to spend the day with the Maynards at home, meet their other children, and take down their story. I had contacted them after a resident at the hospital showed me the blog that Rich and Traci had maintained during Erika's illness. It was informed and reflective, chronicling Erika's progress and setbacks, as well as their own struggles—both to sort out the right course for Erika and to come to terms with its impact on them and the other children. One reason they agreed to talk to me is that they thought their experience might be helpful to other families in their position. I think they're right.

Rich and Traci, both thirty-five, are an exceptionally attractive couple—Traci is slender and pretty; Rich is tall and athletic—and almost improbably middle-American. They were raised in the Illinois town of Aledo, population 3,700, across the river about thirty miles from Muscatine. "We met in preschool," Traci said, and Rich chimed in, "and always kind of had feelings for each other." They began to date in high school—one imagines them as their school's golden couple—then went off together to North-ern Illinois University, about an hour west of Chicago, and were married before graduation in 1993. Traci's degree is in elementary education and Rich's in nursing, and they spent the next three years working in Rockford, Illinois, before moving to Nashville, Tennessee, where Rich completed his training as a nurse-anesthetist and where both Emma and Erika were born.

The Maynards are deeply religious. Traci was raised Catholic, Rich a Methodist, but faith became more central to their lives after they discovered the Willow Creek Com-munity Church outside of Chicago while they were in col-lege. Willow Creek is the best known of America's new breed of megachurches and is the hub of the Willow Creek

Association, comprising some 11,000 like-minded ministries throughout the world. The Maynards' Calvary Church, a hangar-size building in a nearby shopping mall, is an association member. Willow Creek and its fellow churches preach a nondenominational Christianity organized around a few basics—the truth of the Bible, the reality of heaven and hell, a purposeful God, and a path to salvation worked out more or less tête-à-tête with Christ.

God is a palpable presence in the Maynards' blog and in their conversations about Erika. Rich is trained in science, and they are both sophisticated, educated people. But as Rich said, in trying to discern what was best for Erika, their responsibility "was to find out the facts, and make informed decisions, at the same time trusting in God's guidance." Their faith has been an important source of support after the loss of Erika, but in some ways, particularly for Traci, faith has made it harder. They were already resigned to the inevitability of their little girl's death when they discovered the program at Columbia-Presbyterian. It was everything they had been searching for, and their skies grew very bright. Then just as good news was coming from the OR, and they were emailing friends and relatives that it looked like Erika was going to make it, God seemed to turn cruel.

The last few years had been very tough. Rich and Traci did not even know that their daughter had an irreversibly damaged heart until the spring of 2005, barely a year before the surgery. But there had been shadows over Erika almost from the start. A mid-pregnancy alphafetal protein test had been positive, indicating possible chromosomal problems. Erika went full-term, but in the last week of the pregnancy Traci became alarmed when the baby's activity seemed to fall off. Tests showed problematic heart rhythms, and the doctors went right to a C-section. Erika emerged blue, the umbilical cord around her neck, with a strong presence of meconium. Meconium is a baby's first stool. It is usually not evacuated until after birth, but is sometimes released in the womb, especially during a stressful delivery. It is sterile, but if a gasping baby inhales it, it can damage the lungs. Erika was resuscitated, and since she appeared to have inhaled meconium, was transferred to a neonatal intensive care unit. With extra oxygen and antibiotics, however, she did fine, and in about a week her much-relieved parents could bring her home. Erika had experienced heartbeat irregularities in the NICU, however, and sometimes seemed to have trouble breathing. Rich remembers asking one of the doctors whether they should do an echocardiogram. The answer was "No, those symptoms were consistent with meconium aspiration, no need to multiply tests."

At first, everything went well. Erika was a small baby, only four pounds eight ounces at birth, but on Traci's "high-octane breast milk," as her pediatrician called it, she seemed to thrive, gaining weight, a pleasant, happy baby. Then more shadows. At about two months, Erika started to have trouble feeding, difficulty "latching on," Traci said. (Only much later did they realize she may have been struggling for oxygen.) There were signs of oral-motor issues, and she started to lose weight. They ran through one dietary regimen after the other. Nothing seemed to help, and Erika was just barely getting by nutritionally. A genetic workup at Vanderbilt didn't disclose any obvious problems. Since Rich was working in a Nashville-area hospital and had good ties to the Vanderbilt Medical Center, they were far better plugged into the medical system than most couples. But the best the doctors came up with was a generic "failure to thrive."

Sunshine broke through in the spring of 2003, when Erika was almost a year and a half old. First, Rich got an offer to join the anesthesiology practice in Muscatine. Iowa is one of a number of medically underserved states that allow nurse-anesthetists to practice independently, subject to only modest limitations. It was just the kind of practice Rich was looking for. He knew and liked the people, it was prosperous, serving two regional hospitals, the commute was short and would allow more time for Rich to be home. Even more important, the move brought them back within their family network. Erika's slow deterioration, the to-ing and fro-ing between experts, the mysteriousness of it all, was taking a toll. "We were stressed out," Rich said; "in survival mode," Traci added. Muscatine also meant two sets of grandparents a half hour away, and all four were healthy, relatively young, and had known each other since Rich and Traci were kids.

And then they seemed to find the answer. A Vanderbilt doctor had suggested a "G-tube," a feeding tube inserted surgically into the stomach for supplementary feeding. They had been reluctant to try it in Nashville, but after they settled in Muscatine and had the recommendation reinforced by the pediatricians at the University of Iowa, they agreed to try it. Erika not only tolerated the procedure well, but she blossomed. She began to gain weight, Rich said. "She was happier, and that took so much pressure off. She was fine and loving, and life was pretty good." "She was a little delayed in oral motor skills," Traci said, "especially in chewing and swallowing, but there are exercises for that. It was fine." The summer of 2003 was a very good time: Emma and Erika were happy children; Rich and Traci were surrounded by family and friends; the practice was doing well.

It lasted until August. "Erika and I were out in the yard, kind of playing," Rich said. "Emma and Traci were on the other side of the house. Erika suddenly looked up at me and got this really scared look in her eyes. I picked her up and said, 'You okay?' And then she went into a full-blown seizure. She arched her back and got real rigid. She didn't thrash or anything, just tensed up, and got ghostly white, like her heart had stopped, and I'm trying to feel a pulse, and I'm freaking out, and I'm calling, 'Traci, we've got to get her to a hospital.' "

"I called 911," Traci said. "Yes, you called them," Rich said. "I was in denial. Then all of a sudden she stopped breathing and was as pale as could be. It was horrible. I shook her, then held her head close to my ear to see if she was breathing, and then I heard her take a breath. And then she takes a second breath. I laid her down and watched her, and she starts to come around, and in maybe thirty seconds she opened her eyes. And then she was kind of clingy, so we held her for probably fifteen minutes, and then she wanted to get down and go play again, as if nothing had happened." "Most of the seizures were like that," Traci said, although almost never as severe. The first one, Rich believes, was an actual cardiac arrest; just one other one, he thinks, more than two years later, was as bad.

Kids have seizures. Rich talked to the emergency room doctor at the hospital—it was a Sunday—and he said that as long as she'd recovered there was nothing to do but watch her and get a thorough pediatric checkup the next day. Rich had seen "low perfusion" seizures that result from insufficient blood getting to the brain and thought that Erika's seizure looked something like those. In fact, he had hit the nail on the head. But all the pediatricians they talked to over the next couple of years said, "No, this looks like a childhood seizure"—which was also true.

As the seizures continued over the next few weeks, the Maynards consulted with a neurologist. EEGs showed some "seizure activity," but nothing major—she wasn't epileptic, for instance. At the end of September 2003, Erika was put on a mild anticonvulsant, which seemed to ease the seizures somewhat. Rich guesses that she may have had 100 to 150 seizures, or more than one a week, the rest of her life. Although they varied in severity, most were relatively brief, and they tended to bunch, so there were still extended periods without seizure activity. But just as Rich and Traci would start to relax, there'd be another seizure. Eventually, she was labeled as having "complex partial cluster seizures," more of a description, perhaps, than a diagnosis.

The family adjusted. Between seizures, Erika seemed a normal, in most ways a delightful, child. She was funny, loved her family, loved music—Bono and the Calvary Church songs in equal measure—was a great dancer, and had that traffic-stopping smile. But she was also oddly fragile. She was easily upset, and upsets could trigger seizures. Rich and Traci learned about emotional tiptoeing. But this was okay. Kids have seizures and then they outgrow them. And, they told themselves, we are very blessed, with Emma and Erika, our lovely house, our friends, our parents, and our faith.

Over the next year, Erika's vulnerability became more and more apparent. She easily caught respiratory infections and was becoming a regular at the University of Iowa hospital in Iowa City, about forty minutes west of Muscatine. She was hospitalized for pneumonia in the spring of 2004, was diagnosed with asthma that winter, and the following May was in the hospital again with pneumonia. Rich was increasingly convinced that he was seeing perfusion seizures—the rapid heartbeat, pale face, clammy extremities. When the brain is getting insufficient blood, it protects itself by flooding the heart with neurostimulants and shutting down peripheral systems. But all the specialists he spoke to said, "No that's what childhood seizures look like too."

Then he and Traci began to notice that Erika was taking subtle little breaks from play activity—just dropping out for brief periods to catch her breath—and was having more trouble keeping up with Emma. Finally, in January 2005, at a routine assessment of her speech and feeding progress at the University of Iowa's children's hospital, Traci spoke of their worries about the constant colds, the decline in Erika's exercise tolerance, and the continued seizures. The doctors agreed that Erika should be referred for a pulmonary and cardiology workup.

"It took a while to get the joint heart-lung exam scheduled," Traci said. "It wasn't anyone's fault. But it's hard to coordinate two specialists, especially if you're not already a patient. So they didn't happen until April 19. By then, I was full-term with Evan, and the C-section was scheduled for the twenty-first. But I could get around all right, and Rich's mother, Mary, and I took Erika out for the appointment." Erika in the meantime had seemed to be getting better, to the point where Rich and Traci had almost stopped worrying that she might have a heart problem.

Erika "behaved beautifully" during the tests. But Traci and Mary found it alarming that the technician insisted that doctors come in and look at the echocardiogram images even before he finished. Then, when all the tests were completed, the doctors tried to explain gently to Traci that Erika had a very serious heart problem, and there was no treatment for it except a transplant. But because of another condition in her lungs, they did not believe she would be eligible for a transplant. "In other words," Traci said, "she was going to die and there was nothing they could do. I was two days from giving birth, and they're telling me that Erika's going to die, and there was no help for it!" "Traci called me at work," Rich said, "and I could barely understand what she was saying. It didn't make sense. She was just sobbing and sobbing and telling me that Erika was going to die."

Erika had cardiomyopathy. The muscle cells of her heart, the togglelike myoctes that are the engines of the heart's ticktock pumping action, were slowly dying. In the elderly, cardiomyopathy is often a last-stage heart disease, what doctors mean when they talk about "chronic heart failure." A small percentage of children, more often girls, are born with it, and childhood cardiomyopathy usually progresses much faster than cardiomyopathy in adults.

There are palliative treatments, but the only "cure" is a transplant.

But Erika also suffered from pulmonary hypertension. To understand what that means, consider what an astonishing organ the lung is. Every minute, the heart's powerful left ventricle drives more than a gallon of blood through the entire body. But during the same time period, the much weaker right ventricle must drive the same volume of blood through the lungs. That is possible only because the lungs are densely vascularized and maintain an extraordinarily low blood pressure, normally about one-sixth that in the rest of the body. If your normal systolic/diastolic blood-pressure reading is 120/60, your pulmonary blood pressure should be about 20/10. Erika's was as much as five times too high.

Dr. Linda Addonizio, a comfortable grandmotherly woman who heads the pediatric heart transplant section at Columbia-Presbyterian, drew a chart for me. Erika's pulmonary hypertension was "secondary" to her cardiomyopathy. The original cardiomyopathy, she believed, was in the left ventricle. As the weakened ventricular walls strained to keep up with their pumping load, they thickened and stiffened, increasing resistance to the blood flowing in from the lungs. In response, the blood vessels in the lungs tightened up too, increasing pulmonary pressures, the better to resist pushback from the heart. And now the right ventricle had to work harder to get blood *into* the lungs, and the dreadful downward spiral was under way—both ventricles straining, thickening, and stiffening, and the pressures within the lungs steadily rising. At one point, Erika had a pulmonary pressure reading that was actually higher than in the rest of her body. Erika was clearly a very poor candidate for a heart transplant. A heart, after all, is a precious resource. Give Erika a new heart, and those massive pressures within her lungs would destroy it.

After dropping their bombshell on Traci, the doctors, in a sudden fit of common sense, suggested that they put the matter on hold until after the new baby was born— at least as best as Rich and Traci could. In the meantime, the doctors would do more research on Erika's condition. Evan's birth took place on schedule and was otherwise uneventful.

When they reconvened at the end of May, Erika's case had been taken over by Dr. Heather Bartlett, head of the pediatric transplant service at Iowa. She explained that Erika's problem was extremely challenging but not hopeless. Her current lung pressures were indeed too high for a transplant, but there were medications that might bring them down to transplantable ranges.* She recommended starting with Viagra (which was originally developed as a vasodilator). In the meantime, Erika was hospitalized with another bout of pneumonia, so it was summer before her new medication routines were stabilized. They seemed to help. Her oxygen saturation levels were up, her exercise

---

*In theory, Erika's problem might also have been solved with a transplant of a new heart *and* lungs. Heart-lung transplants in adults had been common for a while in the 1980s, but are quite rare now—one recipient is using up a lot of organs. The number of pediatric heart-lung transplants, ever, is fewer than a dozen, and results were generally poor. Doctors mentioned it from time to time, but it was never considered a realistic option.

tolerance was better, she seemed happier. Rich and Traci remember the summer of 2005 as a "good period."

The bad news came in the fall. Yes, the drugs seemed to be helping her breathing, but it was purely palliative. If anything, her lung pressures were even higher, and the course of the cardiomyopathy was accelerating. Bartlett had originally told the Maynards that Erika might have three or four more years to live, but now she feared that a crisis might come much sooner than that. The complexity of Erika's case had also become more than the team in Iowa was prepared to deal with. There was a top pulmonary hypertension specialist at Washington University in St. Louis, however, a Dr. David Balzer, and Bartlett suggested that they try him.

The family made the pilgrimage to St. Louis, about four and a half hours away by car. Erika was just turning four. Balzer's team kept her overnight for another round of heart-lung workups. When they were finished, Balzer agreed with Iowa that Erika could not yet be considered a heart transplant candidate, but suggested a much more aggressive medication regimen—infusing a powerful drug, remodulin, directly into Erika's lungs from an external pump. Erika would have to wear a backpack containing the pump and the drug supply, while the infusion access would be through a permanent access line in her chest. As its name implied, the drug had shown some efficacy in "remodeling" a hypertensive lung—that is, the lung would adapt to the prolonged infusion of pressure-reducing medication by readjusting its own pressure profile, just as it had done in the opposite direction in response to ventricular resistance. The Maynards were cautious. It sounded fairly radical, and they were worried about compromising the quality of Erika's life. In the meantime, however, Erika would add a cardiac-function booster to her drug regime and would be kept on oxygen at night.

Events made up the Maynards' minds. In November, Erika had two dreadful seizures a week apart, both at home. The first culminated in full-blown cardiac arrest. Rich was there and administered CPR. The second was just as bad; at one point Rich thought she was dying. By this time, Rich and Traci were becoming resigned to the knowledge that Erika's options were running out. They'd take their chances with St. Louis.

When the Maynards returned to St. Louis at the end of the month, Balzer and his team not only placed the drug backpack, but also cut a small shunt, or slit, in the wall, or septum, that separated Erika's left and right atria. Balzer cut the shunt with a catheter-based tool threaded through Erika's leg, so there was only a Band-Aid–sized incision. Fixing "atrial septal defects" is a bread-and-butter procedure for congenital surgeons. The danger of a leaky atrial septum is that unoxygenated blood entering the right atrium from the venous system can mix with the oxygenated blood flowing into the left atrium from the lungs. In Erika's case, the doctors were actually creating the leak— if the right ventricle was struggling to get blood into the lungs, some of the backup would be vented away, relieving the atrial pressure and perhaps also maintaining volumes on the left side. Easing the pressures within the heart might accelerate the hoped-for lung remodeling. Balzer also confirmed Rich's suspicion that Erika's seizures had been low-perfusion seizures, and he made it clear that Erika was already into the end stages of her disease. Another major seizure could be fatal, and the septal shunt itself was a desperate measure. If the remodulin therapy didn't work within a few months, there would be little hope for her.

It took a few days to tune Erika's medications, but by the end of the first week, Erika appeared to be tolerating the remodulin beautifully, and had no trouble with the backpack. It weighed only a pound and a half, and she wore it all day except in the bath. As Traci and Rich became more accustomed to the machinery, Traci replaced the black hospital pack with ones in Erika's favorite pinks and lavenders. I saw a home video of Erika scurrying with other kids at a church Sunday school program, apparently happy and normal, her little pink backpack coordinated with a white shirt and pink slacks, and looking like nothing other than a handy place for a favorite toy.

The next couple of months went very well. Erika clearly felt better, and her play energy noticeably improved. There was a bump in the road in January, when she had another extended siege at the Iowa University children's hospital—starting with pneumonia, as before, but topped off by a nasty viral lung infection. Heather Bartlett told Rich and Traci that Erika had no reserves left—she was "one cold, one flu season, one cough away from a catastrophic illness." By now, they were focused on a transplant as the only remaining option. That depended entirely on the success of the remodulin therapy in lowering Erika's pulmonary pressures, but there were multiple signs that the drugs were working. As Erika recovered from her illnesses, she bounced right back and often seemed almost like her old self.

At the end of March 2006, however, the long-circling shadows suddenly engulfed them—or so it seemed. Another round of tests in St. Louis showed that there had been no remodeling effect in Erika's lungs. The drug infusions made her feel better, but the hypertension was even worse than in the fall. Erika was not a candidate for a transplant and, as far as St. Louis could tell, was not likely to become one. On their blog, Rich and Traci posted the news for their friends and family—the doctors' conclusions were "a really awful indication of things to come." The blog went on:

> She's still energetic and playful. Pretty happy. No signs of pain or fear. She really has no idea that anything is wrong with her little body. We're relieved that she is able to be at home on our own terms as opposed to being cooped up in a hospital somewhere. We continue to focus on the day-to-day things and not look too far into the future. . . . Please pray for Erika's happiness and disposition. No pain, no fear. Pray for Emma and Evan and various aspects of this situation that are affecting them or will affect them eventually. And pray for strength for Traci and me as we move forward. As always, thank you for caring.
>   Rich and Traci

Out of the Blue

In the first weeks after the terrible news from St. Louis, the Maynards concentrated on adjusting to their fate. Erika was in fairly good shape, still bouncy and smiling on the home videos, although the seizures were becoming more frequent. The doctors' best guess was that she had six months to two years to live, but the Maynards counted on less than that. Realistically, once school started in the fall, she couldn't be quarantined from Emma and Emma's friends, and was bound to catch the childhood bug that would finish her. "We drew a lot of support from our families and a few close friends," Traci said. "We were at peace with whatever was going to happen." Rich added, "We just wanted to give Erika a good summer."

At the same time, they kept in touch with Web-based support groups for parents of children with problems like Erika's. Chat groups traded names of experts, and two cardiologists specializing in childhood pulmonary hypertension were always at the top of the list—a Dunbar Ivy in Denver and a Robyn Barst at Columbia-Presbyterian. They decided to email them both, mostly, in Rich's words, "to see if there was anything else to do to help her before—before her death." The email summarized Erika's condition and asked if they would be willing to look at her records.

They got a reply from Barst within about twenty minutes. Linda Addonizio had been with Barst when it came in, and they both drafted it. They made no promises, but, yes, they would like to see the records. And a couple of weeks later, the Maynards got another email: "We think it would be worth your time to come out here."

From the Maynards' blog, an entry by Traci:

Maybe it was just a coincidence that she responded so quickly, but I choose to think of it as a "God thing."

Anyway, we feel the door of opportunity was opened for us. We are planning to drive out to NYC, since we can't fly due to Erika's condition, on Mother's Day, May 14. We will take two days to travel, with time to get settled before our first appt on Tuesday, May 16. We do know they have Erika scheduled for a heart cath on Thursday. We will plan to head home on Friday, God willing.

I know God wants what is best for all of us, and I'm coming to a better place to accept whatever God's will is. Please pray for our safe travels, Erika's strength to endure this big trip, the heart cath to go smoothly, the results to be favorable, our other 2 (Emma and Evan) to get along well with their grandparents, and for Rich and me to be able to accept whatever they discover and be able to rise above our circumstance and press on.

When they arrived at the hospital on Tuesday, instead of visiting with Barst as they expected, they were given a schedule for a full day of tests. To their surprise, they realized they were undergoing a full transplant evaluation. "We were seeing a psychologist," Rich said. On Wednesday, when they met both Barst and Addonizio in turn, they were impressed with their thorough mastery of Erika's history.

Addonizio had come to Columbia-Presbyterian in 1984 with the express intention of creating better treatment alternatives for kids with pulmonary hypertension, and told me that they were still "about the only place" that routinely transplants them. She is the transplant specialist, while Barst is the expert on pulmonary hypertension.

"Linda told us that they had successfully transplanted children with higher pulmonary pressures than Erika's," Rich said. "And she thought that if Erika's numbers were close to what they were in St. Louis that they would be inclined to transplant, which kind of blew us away. I mean, we were like, Wow! She might have a chance. It all depended on the cath readings on Thursday."

Pulmonary hypertension is measured by inserting a catheter-based sensor into the heart. The index scale, known as the PVR, for "pulmonary vascular resistance," sets a value of 2 as approximately normal. Erika's last PVR had been about 12, or the same as normal pressure in the rest of her body. The PVR ceiling for heart transplants had traditionally been as low as 3, but the surgeons told me that they had recently been taking cases as high as 6. When I asked Addonizio about those limits, she waved them away. "I love our surgeons," she said, "but the great majority of their cases are adults, where wide-sweeping formulae like that make sense. But kids are very different, and much less predictable. Erika was very similar to a boy we'd done who had PVRs much higher than she did." She gave me a preliminary copy of an article documenting dozens of her unit's successful pediatric transplants in cases with very high PVRs.

The next two days, Wednesday and Thursday, were difficult ones for Erika, and punctuated by two seizures. But they still managed to finish the full run of tests. On Thursday, while Erika was in the cath lab, Rich and Traci talked through their options—were they willing to try a transplant? One of the purposes of the cath, besides getting a new baseline PVR, was to assess her reactivity to medications. Rich said they finally decided that "if she comes back with a PVR in the 5-to-6, maybe up to the 7, range, and they want to do a transplant, we felt we really ought to do it. But if it comes back higher than that, we're not going to put her through it. We're not going to take the chance.

"And then they brought Erika back and Dr. [Diane] Kerstein, the cardiologist who did the reactivity testing, came into the room and was really upbeat. She said it started off really bad, the pressures were very high. But with the right combination of medicines, they'd gotten her down to 1.7. We were just floored. Oh, my God. With all our support systems praying. . . ."

Traci said, "We felt that we were on the verge of this miracle, that God had opened his doors wide for us to proceed forward." "We were thinking, How could we not do this?" Rich added. They posted the news on their blog:

> We are simply overjoyed. God has given us exactly what we asked for. We prayed intently that God would either take her now, without pain and suffering, or bring her through a transplant without significant complications or problems. We also prayed that our path ahead would be pretty clear and that we would not be forced to make a difficult decision if the cath results were borderline. We know she still has a long road ahead, but we are encouraged to know that God is listening to and answering our prayers.

If there was to be a transplant, the doctors told them, it should be sooner, not later. The Maynards could go home for a few weeks if they wanted more time to pre-

pare, or they could check Erika into the unit now so they
could start the listing process. Addonizio also told them
that Erika would do fine with the St. Louis unit, if they
preferred to be closer to home. They thought hard about
going home, but decided not to take the chance. Erika had
had three seizures since their arrival in New York. It
wasn't clear she could even survive the trip to Iowa, and
the Columbia-Presbyterian team was clearly deep and
experienced. They would stay. Erika was admitted that
night, and given a 1A listing by the pediatric transplant
committee the next morning. Jonathan Chen, who represented Surgery at the meeting, said she was viewed as "a
very high-risk case" but not outside the range of cases they
had successfully transplanted in the past.

Then the waiting began. The Maynards were in a hotel
across the George Washington Bridge in New Jersey, just
fifteen minutes from the hospital. Rich's parents, who had
been looking after Emma and Evan, were driving out to
join them. Erika, who had spent a lot of time in hospitals,
was making new friends. "Everyone says how cute she is
and they love her pink flip-flops," Traci posted.

Erika was approved by the transplant committee on Friday, May 19. During that weekend, the whole next week,
and the Memorial Day weekend, there was nothing to be
done except wait. Rich's parents arrived with Emma and
Evan on Saturday, although his father returned home on
Monday. Erika had several stress-induced seizures early in
her stay, but the staff quickly learned how to avoid trig-
gering them. But she was kept in the pediatric ICU because
the powerful medication she was getting could trigger
seizures by itself. She also had a bad day when a midweek

exam requiring fasting was inordinately delayed, upsetting her enough that Rich and Traci stayed with her overnight. The rest of the time she seemed to be thriving. Most days the whole family stayed with Erika, but with beautiful weather and Rich's mom, Mary, available to spell them, Rich and Traci ventured into "the Huge Apple" as Emma called it—the first trip for all of them. They learned to use the subway, took the kids to Central Park, and began to worry about money. And they guiltily recorded the frisson of excitement when television flashed news of a traffic accident that left a young boy in a coma. On the Memorial Day weekend, Rich's two sisters arrived to replace Mary on the relay team, and Rich flew home on Monday to catch up at work, with plans to return on Friday.

The next week went very well for Erika as she continued to settle into the hospital, but the strain of waiting was beginning to tell on everyone else. Then, just before 4 A.M. on Friday, June 2, Traci posted on the blog:

Dear family & friends

Please pray. I just got off the phone with one of our cardiologists, Dr. Hsu. She is part of the transplant team. She said they MAY have a donor for Erika. She said it is too early to be sure, however, they plan to get things started with Erika around 9 am. I'm shaking with so much fear and joy. Please, please, pray for the donor family and for Erika.

Rich had planned to fly back to New York that night. Instead, he'd catch the early plane along with Traci's mother and would land at 11:15. At 11:22, Traci posted:

I signed the consent for the transplant. I'm very emotional, but trying to be calm for Erika. They will come for her in 10 minutes. Please be praying. The transplant should last 4 to 6 hours.

The Transplant

I had arranged with the transplant team to observe an operation, and got the call for the Maynard surgery at about 10 A.M. "Skin time" about noon, I was told, but was warned that the start time would likely slip. I was happy that it was a pediatric case. Even better, it was in the daytime. Jan Quaegebeur was the pediatric surgeon on rotation, and the nurses had reassured Traci that he was "the best of the best," someone with whom they'd trust their own children.

Erika was brought in about 12:15. She was fussing, but the women in the room surrounded her, cooing soothingly. Johanna Schwarzenberger, the anesthesiologist, got a line in, and Erika was asleep within a minute or so. Besides Schwarzenberger, there was Daphne Hsu, from Addonizio's team of transplant cardiologists; Rozelle Corda, the surgical assistant; and the two nurses.

Schwarzenberger introduced me to Hsu, who explained the nature of Erika's cardiomyopathy (a "frustrating disease," she called it, because there was no therapy except a transplant) as well as the difficulties posed by the pulmonary hypertension. She told me that Quaegebeur had ordered a right ventricular assist device, an RVAD, to be on standby in case the new heart needed temporary help pushing against the lung pressures. I had never before seen a cardiologist in the OR. I later mentioned that to Addonizio, who smiled and said: "We always do that. The parents go through this terrible buildup to the transplant, then they sit and wait for hours with no information. It's only right that a doctor is there who can come out and give them updates from time to time." A lovely touch—perhaps one of the benefits of a primarily female practice group.

Quaegebeur came by from time to time to check on Erika's prep work and the progress of the organ. Unusually, it was coming from a town in southern Canada, and the harvest team had earlier reported that it was a "good heart"—it was the right weight for Erika, and the donor had died suddenly, without any intimations of heart disease. The noon schedule for bringing Erika to the OR assumed that the plane would land at Teterboro at about 1:00. We finally heard from the harvest team about 1:30, but they were just leaving Canada, with an ETA at the hospital of about 2:45.

Because of the importance of limiting an organ's cold ischemic time, standard practice is to "explant" the old heart before the new one arrives. Quaegebeur, who seemed in an unusually democratic mood, asked the team when he should start the surgery. The collective decision was that it should be at 2:10, assuming that it would take him twenty-five minutes to get Erika on bypass and maybe ten minutes to remove her heart. A nurse came by to report a heavy thunderstorm outside, and the likelihood of flying delays.

Quaegebeur scrubbed and gowned and started operating at just about 2:10, working with his usual unhurried speed and without an assistant surgeon, as he seems to prefer. By my watch, it took him thirteen minutes to get Erika on bypass and four to complete the explant. The heart, which was about the size of a lamb's, was put into a white plastic bowl and removed to a table off to the side of the room. Some minutes later, glancing in that direction, I suppressed a gasp. A young woman in a white lab coat who must have entered the OR during the explant was busy slicing up Erika's heart and placing the pieces into an array of test tubes. To me, the finality of the procedure was staggering. In ORs, however, cold logic rules. A heart so weak that it needs replacing won't withstand the shock of the explant, so there is no possibility of reversing the operation. If the pathology lab was to glean useful lessons from Erika's heart, the samples had to be as fresh as possible.

There was roughly a forty-minute wait before the harvest team arrived. Erika was resting comfortably on the bypass. Most of the team found places to sit, but Quaegebeur kept his post at the right side of the table, as if he was standing sentry. It was a good opportunity for questions, so I went back to the table. He nodded to me, pointed down at Erika's empty chest, and said, "Isn't that an amazing sight." I asked if he knew anything about the new heart, and he said, "No, and I don't want to. Especially with kids, they always involve some terrible tragedy." Quaegebeur talked about the high pulmonary pressures and the riskiness it added to the operation, and he was pessimistic about the RVAD: "I hope we don't have to go down that road. It might keep her alive for a few weeks, but it's usually just a bridge to nowhere."

Then he walked me through the standard transplant steps. A heart has just four external connecting points, two for inflow and two for outflow. The inflow connections are on the back wall of the chest. The vena cava is a huge vertical pipe that collects the deoxygenated blood, and dumps it into the right atrium through a stubby sidelong T-connector. On the other side of the heart, four veins, two from each lung, feed reoxygenated blood into the left atrium. Instead of severing the veins, Quaegebeur left in place the two rear atrial walls of the old heart with their connections intact. Making the inflow connections would then just be a matter of sewing the back walls of Erika's old heart onto the new one. The outflow connections are even simpler: he would just sew Erika's aorta and pulmonary artery onto their respective openings in the new heart. "So this is not technically difficult?" I asked. "No, not at all," he shrugged. "It's very straightforward."

By my watch, it was 3:12 when the harvest team arrived. The immigration authorities, of all things, had held them up for some fifteen minutes to confirm that it was just a heart in that box, and then they had run into the thunderstorm. But there was no stopping for conversation. As soon as they entered the room, a nurse reached into the ice carrier, pulled out the plastic bag with the new heart, opened it, and put it into a pail at the foot of the table. Quaegebeur pulled out the dripping heart, dried it with the blue towels, then set it next to Erika's chest opening. He removed the big wedge of fat on top, cut out and trimmed the atrial openings, and was executing the transplant within three minutes. He worked steadily and silently, at one point scooping handfuls of ice from the organ bag and dumping it into the chest. At 3:45, he told the perfusionist, Kevin Charette, to start rewarming. At 3:55, he started unclamping, although he was still touching up the stitching—trading the possibility of a little bleeding to get the new heart started as soon as possible. Total ischemic time was 216 minutes, an excellent number, especially given the delays.

It was exciting to see Erika's new heart jitter into life. I can't read EKGs, but I knew that the sharp "R" points register the beats, and there they were! "That looks good, doesn't it?" I asked Schwarzenberger. "No!" she snapped, waving vaguely at one part of the pattern that was "much too rounded." She was about to get very busy.

Balkiness is common in a newly transplanted heart. The little clump of muscle and tubing that Quaegebeur had just sewn into Erika's chest had suffered through a day of savage abuse. The brain death of its original owner unleashed a cataclysmic flood of chemicals that, in Craig Smith's words, signaled all the other organs "that they should line up and die as fast as they could." The self-inflicted injuries from the first few minutes after brain death are a major reason most transplants fail after twelve years or so.* And that initial cascade of insults is grossly compounded by the transplant team—chopping the heart out of its owner's chest, flooding it with cardioplegia and

---

*Children who get transplants therefore need one or more additional transplants to survive into adulthood. It is not because the new heart doesn't grow. A baby who gets another baby's heart will reach his teens with a teenage heart, but one that is already failing.

other chemicals, then plunging it into an ice chest. That a transplanted heart wakes up at all is astonishing, not that it wakes up crankily.

To help reacclimate a transplanted heart, you can ease it back into service with the bypass machine. After watching Erika's new heart struggle for several minutes, Quaegebeur reset the bypass cannulae, and he and Charette restarted the machine. This time, there was no cross-clamp, so Erika would be perfused by *both* her new heart and the machine. Flooded with fresh blood, and with minimum work to do, a new heart should get back to something like its old self in a quarter hour or so.

Over the next hour, Erika was weaned off the bypass machine three times, by my count, and each time they had to put her back on. It was expected that the right ventricle would struggle, since it had to push against those heavy pulmonary pressures. Much more alarming, the left ventricle seemed to be "resting" in Schwarzenberger's words. Its unassisted ejection fraction was only 26 percent, a level usually associated with chronic heart failure patients. The air of concern around the table was palpably rising.

Then Quaegebeur did one of the most intelligent things I've seen a surgeon do. "I'm going to take a break," he announced. "We'll give her a good run with the bypass and see what happens." But he was clearly upset, and as he was leaving, he told me: "I think it's the new heart. We never know the whole story of what these organs go through. But the left ventricle isn't responding. This was always a difficult case, but I never expected *this*."

After Quaegebeur left, the room was very quiet. Erika was a mound of blue towels with a bowled-shaped opening at top, envined with tubing and holding a beating heart. Kevin Charette, who had to keep his post at the bypass machine, and I were the only males in the room. My back was hurting, so I found a chair off to the side, but the women formed a ring around Erika. They stood silently for a while, then quietly began to chat. The scene was oddly peaceful, and for the moment at least, Erika seemed very safe.

Quaegebar returned after about forty minutes, looking refreshed. He regowned quickly, and everyone took their places. For almost an hour, they worked on coaxing Erika off the bypass. Finally, Quaegebeur shook his head and said, "I'm sorry. I think this is insoluble." The room was silent. He waited a bit, then said, "What would you like me to do?" I heard two or three voices say, "You said you wanted the RVAD." Quaegebeur nodded—"Okay." Allison Cohen relieved Charette at the bypass machine, and he went off to fetch the RVAD.

Charette returned with another worker, pushing a refrigerator-sized machine on heavy wheels, with a foliage of cannulae like the bypass machine's. It took about a half hour to make the hookup. RVADs are infrequently resorted to, and Charette carefully reviewed the connection sequences with Quaegebeur before they started. The RVAD would intercept most of the blood coming from the vena cava and pump it directly into the pulmonary artery, bypassing both the right atrium and the right ventricle. I was a bit puzzled that they were using an RVAD, since the left ventricle seemed to be the main problem. Addonizio later explained that, with sluggishness in the left ventricle, the pressures in Erika's lungs were increasing, placing even greater stress on the new heart's already-struggling right ventricle. Easing the load on the right ventricle with the RVAD would allow more time for the left ventricle to work out its problems.

With the protruding RVAD cannulae, Erika's chest could not be closed in the usual way, so Quaegebeur taped a sterile plastic cover over the opening. Infection risk was obviously high, but there was no alternative. I stayed in the OR until a transport team arrived to convey poor Erika and her whole rumbling train of equipment to her new home in the intensive care unit.

Purgatory

All the cardiothoracic office staff and nurses knew about "the little girl" and followed her case, most of them praying for her daily. Diane Amato, the division administrator, kept me informed by email—some days things were looking up, some days not. I saw Quaegebeur at meetings a couple of times, and he was quite pessimistic. "I hate to think of what we're putting those poor parents through," he said on one occasion.

Rich and Traci kept their family, friends, and church connections informed on their blog. Their first posting after the surgery came about 9 P.M. that night:

Erika has been back in her room for a couple of hours now. She is very critical. Literally, moment to moment. Blood pressure is low, but she continues to make urine which indicates that her brain is being adequately perfused. The doctors are not optimistic about her pulling through this, but we know that God is in control. We have made it clear to the team that we believe there are certainly worse things than death, and when they feel that enough is enough, then we can rest with that. You should know that one of the reasons we elected to stay in NYC and pursue a heart transplant was because of the fact that Erika was so sick. Over the past several weeks we had come to suspect that she might not make it through the summer, let alone the year. We have no regrets about the decision to pursue the transplant. We're sure we'll have plenty of time to think about it in the days to come. We need your prayers now more than ever. Keeping the faith and still trusting in the supreme authority of God—let His will be done.

The surgery was on a Friday, June 2. Rich posted after midnight that evening.

This night of horror continues, and Erika is hanging in there. I feel I have a little better handle on what's going on physiologically. There is still reason to have some hope tonight. Erika's heart will either fail completely, or it will gradually strengthen/hypertrophy against the high pulmonary resistance. Meanwhile she's been bleeding quite a bit from around the RVAD and has received 2 units of blood and other blood products to slow the bleeding. The bleeding does seem to be slowing down, and they'll keep giving volume and blood products until her new heart gets better or worse. Erika is being sedated heavily. Traci and I are taking turns talking to her to let her know we're here with her and love her. I was encouraged when she responded to me with a twitch of arms and a little bit of a nod immediately after I asked her if she wanted to go swing. She loves to swing. Please pray that that new little heart of hers will take off and work like it's supposed to.

The rest of the night was even worse. At about 11 A.M., the next morning, Rich posted:

Our little Erika is hanging in there. The surgery team removed some clots from around her heart and placed a ventricular pacing wire. Her pressure has been up a little higher ever since. We're taking this hour to hour.

Erika seemed to improve a bit the rest of Saturday. Traci posted late Saturday night:

I must admit, I have spent the last 36 hours emotionally overwhelmed. We are in the midst of the fight of our lives. Please pray for the pressures in her lungs to decrease and the pumping of her beautiful new heart to become stronger with each beat. She continues to become more stable as time passes. Praise God! Much love and appreciation.

Sunday was a good day. Erika seemed to be stabilizing. Both sets of grandparents and several aunts and uncles had joined Rich and Traci, and they brought Emma and Evan to the hospital to visit their parents. By Monday, the left ventricle was improving, but the right ventricle wasn't yet strong enough on its own to come off the RVAD. She continued under heavy sedation and was receiving stupendous cocktails of medications. On Tuesday, Traci posted that Erika had had a rough night, but a medication adjustment had seemed to stabilize her again. The hospital arranged a meeting between Emma and a child psychologist to help her process what was going on. Traci concluded her last post of the day:

> I would be telling you a half-truth, if I didn't mention the heartache we feel watching our sweet Erika go through all of this. She does appear comfortable, for which we are thankful. I understand God knows the bigger picture and only wants what is absolutely the best for His children whom He loves so incredibly much. It isn't always easy to feel thankful, but when I start to feel myself sinking, I try to journal all that I am thankful for in that day. As one of my very best friends has said, "Just hold on."

On Wednesday afternoon, Rich posted:

> We have some good news to report. Erika's right ventricle is working! It's weak, and needs more time to come around, but it's working, This is HUGE! Her left ventricle appears to be functioning normally. The transplant docs seem more optimistic about her chances of doing well provided we can prevent new problems from cropping up. Erika is such a strong willed child. She's a fighter, always has been. Anything can happen. That said, I'm starting to like her chances. As always thanks

for your prayers and concern. And thanks be to God for progress.

Thursday morning brought a major reversal, as Erika seemed to fall into a pulmonary hypertensive crisis. The team checked everything—clotting around the heart, her drips, the RVAD—everything looked right. After about a half hour they realized that the night nurse had mixed up Erika's antihypertensive medication with another child's. They had both been given the same drug, but Erika had received only a third of her usual dose. Rich later posted:

This was a substantial setback and it will probably take her several hours to get back to her precrisis level of stability. People make mistakes. Her night nurse has been with Erika for the last 3 nights. She's a great nurse. No hard feelings there. She apologized, she was very emotional. Mistakes happen, Erika is still with us, they intervened appropriately . . . time to move on.

Some months later, he reflected, "In retrospect, things seemed to be going more favorably for Erika prior to this event. I don't think she ever recovered from it." (When I asked Addonizio about it, she just winced.) But Erika was restabilized, and on Friday tolerated a changeover of her RVAD apparatus, a sometimes tricky operation, without incident. Traci posted on Saturday night that Erika's "blood pressure, heart rate and [oxygen] saturation continued to hold steady throughout the day and evening." But she had some bleeding in the afternoon, and with her regimen of blood thinners, bleeding was dangerous. The team had found the problem and fixed it. She went on: "We are struggling to see Erika go through so much. This is exactly what we didn't want to see happen to our little girl."

On Sunday morning, Traci reported that Erika had a "steady night," although there was still some bleeding. The good news was that her pulmonary hypertension was dropping, and the doctors were considering whether to ease back on her medications.

But Erika began bleeding heavily again on Sunday, and "crashed" early Monday morning. Traci posted:

I can't quite understand why she continues to rebound from these episodes. You would think that in this weakened status, it wouldn't take much to push her over the edge. We told Dr. Addonizio that, heart breaking as it is, we are prepared for what may lie right around the corner. Instead, Dr. Addonizio told us that she has seen kids as sick, or sicker than Erika and they walk out of here. We are in such a tough spot. We long to have hope and want to trust God will heal Erika's sick little body, but we also want to be emotionally prepared if He chooses to call her home. Like I've been saying for months, I want to get to a place where I can accept either outcome and be at peace.

Rich posted again late that night:

What an emotional day this has been. The last 48 hours have been very rough. We've basically censored our last couple of entries because the details have been too painful to convey. I didn't want anyone to know what we were willingly subjecting our little girl to. With each unit of blood and each "exploration" our spirits have been progressively crushed. This morning was particularly rough as Traci and I were awakened by the sound of some of the nurses changing the linens beneath Erika. In addition to the bleeding from her chest, it was apparent that she was bleeding from somewhere in her GI tract as well. I got up to have a look and over the next couple of minutes Erika went into a full scale cardiac arrest. It took some time for the medical team's intervention to resolve the problem. This was the last straw. We had a talk with her doctors informing them that we have had enough, and that when they were ready to terminate their efforts to help Erika, we were ok with that. To our surprise, the transplant doc seemed unfazed by the fact that Erika was bleeding so much. She said short of her bleeding into her brain, she was still capable of making a complete recovery. She was not ready to give up.

The next day the surgeons decided they wanted to remove the RVAD, because they thought it was becoming part of Erika's problem. The cardiologists convinced them to wait another day. But on Wednesday, Erika experienced massive bleeding in her lungs, the cumulative effect of the postsurgical regimen of blood-thinning drugs and the RVAD's pushing blood through her lungs' high resistance. The Maynards had had enough. It was left to the junior resident, Mike Bowdish, actually to remove the support systems—"one of the hardest things I've ever had to do," he told me later. But he stayed past his shift to ensure that he would do it—"I wanted her die in peace." Bowdish said he gave her a large dose of pain medication before turning off the drips and pumps: "She died on her own. It was only the drugs and machines that were keeping her alive." Rich and Traci stayed with Erika till the end.

The Maynards posted that night, June 14, twelve days after the surgery:

> It is with great sadness that we write to inform you that our daughter, Erika Kate Maynard has died. We are comforted to know that she is in heaven, singing and dancing with the angels at this time. Erika had a pulmonary hypertensive crisis this afternoon and was unable to recover. She passed at 7:35 P.M. eastern time.

Aftermath

The Maynards were still struggling to come to terms with what had happened when I visited three months later, and Traci was still posting to their blog. One from early September, addressed to "Dear Friends & Family" was particularly sad:

> I must continue to be honest with you. Our life isn't getting easier as time goes on, and I'm not always praising God. The reality of this storm continues to blow us to pieces sometimes. I'm ready for Erika to come home. She's been on "vacation" long enough. I'm angry that God allowed her to be taken from us after 4 1/2 years

of falling in love with one of His most precious gifts. Rich and I revisit the decisions we made and wonder why the doors were open SO WIDE only to lose her in the end. Sometimes we feel betrayed and that our trust has been shattered. I have really tried to be positive and thankful, but sometimes I just don't have that mind set or the energy. I wish I could be strong all the time, but as time marches on, it does present new feelings and new issues to deal with. I'm realizing how rare her condition was and how it seems like few families must endure a loss like we have.

Rich expanded a bit on the feeling of betrayal. When Hsu came out of the OR to tell them about the RVAD and to convey Quaegebeur's doubts, he said: "I was incredulous. I was thinking, it's a God thing, and it couldn't possibly be that we had so much excitement and so much faith that she was going to do well with the transplant. . . . We were emailing everybody back home, and everybody back home was saying 'Erika Maynard is getting her transplant today!' And everybody was flying high." The feeling of betrayal lingered. "We put our faith in God and the transplant team. We realized we were laying it all on the line, but we just felt it was all going to work out. We have at times felt betrayed because God could have delivered her through the whole experience, but didn't."

But they were working on it. Traci said: "Just within the last week I can really say that I'm starting to feel God blessing us and understanding that Erika is in a better place, and that she's not having to suffer here. Because even if the transplant had gone well, she wasn't going to be a healthy, normal child. Death was an inevitable thing for her prematurely. We were going to have to restrict her more and more from the things she loved to do, and she was going to become more and more aware of her differences and her problems."

They also spoke of the "lessons" from their experience, and "Erika's purpose," and I asked them to talk more about that. Traci said, "We've led such blessed lives up until now. And now we've learned to open our eyes to the suffering world, we realize that families are struggling with critically ill children every day, not to mention the balancing act of having other children." Since Erika's diagnosis, the Maynards have become members of a support group for families with critically ill children and through the Web have formed a relationship with a Texas girl who has a problem much like Erika's.

Rich began quietly investigating the community resources that are available to support families through such crises, and late in 2006 filed papers to form the Erika Kate Foundation to "render emotional, spiritual, and financial assistance to families of children with cardiomyopathy, pulmonary hypertension, or who are awaiting a heart transplant." He said he had found a number of "good and talented people" who are interested in the problem.

"Another lesson," Traci said, "is the beauty of simplicity. It doesn't take a trip to Disneyland to be close to your child. With Erika, you couldn't trek across country or go camping, but we could put up a tent in the backyard and eat popcorn, and listen to the bugs chirp. She loved this time together."

She went on: "And going along with the simplicity theme, you realize how society tries to push kids into doing instead of just being, like 'Let's do soccer, let's do dance, let's do, do, do, do, do.' And the more you do the better you are."

Rich added: "We knew Erika's prognosis wasn't good, so we were forced to focus literally on enjoying every day and every moment. And that was a great gift. I've noticed now, even three months later, I don't really want much more. And that might have been one of Erika's purposes—to move us from our comfort zone, the mind-set of acquisition and savings and keeping up with the Joneses. I think it's redirecting us to do something more positive and meaningful, that might make a positive impact on some people's lives. We're trying to breathe in deep so we can go out and make a difference in this messed-up world."

Then Traci said: "And the real gift was just the four and a half years we shared with Erika. We could have easily not had them at all because of all the problems that she had, or could have lost her a lot sooner. We always adjusted, even in the last year. We had a lot of fun together as a family. And we are thankful we didn't spend this past year in the hospital. Erika was able to enjoy her life, without fear, pain, and any knowledge of how sick she was. She definitely had a purpose, and we definitely have a passion to continue her purpose. We're trying the best we can to get through this thing called life." She began crying softly.

Chapter 6

SCHOOL FOR HEART SURGEONS

A DEATH LIKE ERIKA MAYNARD'S REVERBERATES through the cardiothoracic division. Cardiac surgeons see more deaths than surgeons in most other specialties, but the deaths of young people, and of children, are especially hard. Administrative staff who had never seen Erika were aware that she had died. Learning how to deal with death, however, is part of the training for heart surgeons. And since Columbia is a medical school, and the cardiothoracic attendings are university faculty, training is central to what they do.

Graduation

Eric Rose's apartment, a duplex penthouse on a quiet Manhattan side street with a wraparound terrace and a view of the East River, befits the seven-figure income of a chairman of Columbia-Presbyterian's Department of Surgery. Perhaps a hundred people were gathered on a crisp June evening to celebrate Mauricio Garrido's graduation from the cardiothoracic residency program. Rose is a lean, forceful, fifty-five-year-old who has spent his entire post–high school career at Columbia. He was Craig Smith's predecessor as cardiothoracic division chief and is an authority on transplants and heart-assist devices.

Garrido, the beaming guest of honor, seemed as pleased at the prospect of sleeping late the next morning as he was to be a newly minted heart surgeon. Residencies at the cardiothoracic division last for two years. Two new residents are taken in each year, on staggered six-month starts; and on the last six months of a rotation, each resident serves as chief. The chief resident carries the same surgical caseload as his juniors, but does much more of the actual surgery. And since chiefs are also in charge of scheduling, most, as Garrido did, make a point of assigning themselves the most difficult cases, to sop up every possible last chance at learning. The gods of residencies display their special knack for sadism, however, by also giving chiefs control of OR assignments and ICU beds, the most crucial resources in a surgical practice. In a resource-constrained setting like Columbia-Presbyterian, therefore, Garrido constantly found himself in the awkward position of delivering messages such as "Sorry, Craig, you have to cancel your last surgery, I'm giving the room to Mehmet."

Garrido is Cuban-American, and from his blue-ribbon resumé—Cornell engineering degree, Yale medical school, Columbia surgical residency—I assumed he was descended from the island's once-exalted elite. Not at all. He was raised in Union City, New Jersey, in a working-class family—his father was a deliveryman, and often semidisabled with heart disease. The glittering academic record was built by a scholarship boy, with an occasional assist from foundations on the lookout for deserving Hispanic kids. He is grounded, without a hint of swagger, cautious, even a bit plodding, solid through and through, but underneath it all, fiercely competitive. "There is a lot of testosterone around here," he told me. "It's almost a pinnacle of competitiveness—after all, it's New York City, then Columbia-Presbyterian, then surgery, then *heart* surgery."

After the dinner, everyone crowded in from the terraces, and Smith made a short speech celebrating the division's progress and congratulating Garrido, invoking Rocky Marciano's adage that it's the fighter who's fastest to his feet after a knockdown who wins the fight. Garrido thanked everyone, told a few stories, then singled out Mehmet Oz for teaching him that your career is limited only by yourself; Smith for his lessons in clarity, self-discipline, and results; and his father for teaching him that every endeavor, from cooking *arroz con pollo* to heart surgery, has its own art.

Creating Cardiac Surgeons

The content of advanced surgical training is both elaborately specified and quite open-ended. The Accreditation Council for Graduate Medical Education, the primary certification authority, specifies how many and what kind of procedures a resident must participate in over the course of training. The resident enters each operation into a national Web-based reporting system, and final printouts must be signed off by the resident, by Mike Argenziano, the residency program director, and by Smith. Audit teams periodically show up at teaching hospitals, often without notice, to review the quality and content of the program.

The authorities are completely silent, however, on the details of what is actually taught, and the profession wouldn't want it any other way. While there are many textbooks and videos describing a precise way to execute, say, a bypass graft, most surgeons prefer to evolve their own styles. Sherwin Nuland, an author and longtime professor of surgery at Yale University, said, "Surgery is an art form. You have to leave room for individual creativity." Smith told me that he trained under a "Kirklinite"—an acolyte of a famous surgeon, John Kirklin, who had attempted to specify, down to each stitch, how to execute every important procedure. "I can still recite some of those routines by heart," he said. "It got almost robotic. When I first started teaching, I was very specific. But over time I saw how former students had evolved quite different methods, and they all seem to do fine."

But even at Columbia-Presbyterian, there are a few procedures that everyone agrees should be executed uniformly. Placing a bypass cannula in the aorta is at the top of the list. The aortic arch rises straight up from the left ventricle then turns sharply downward, so it is the locus of probably the most violent blood-flow dynamics in the entire body. If the cannula blew out, it would create an unholy, bloody mess, so there is "a Columbia-Presbyterian way" of inserting and anchoring it. It is not the only possible method—Jan Quaegebeur is European-trained and uses a different technique—but it is safe and reliable, and all residents are taught to use it. I asked Smith to think of others, and he came up with just two—placing a retrograde cardioplegia catheter and seating a valve. Both can be tricky, he said, so you might as well learn one method and get good at it—"like practicing scales."

Residents occasionally yearn for greater uniformity. "I'd be working on, say, an aortic root," Garrido said, "and one attending would tell me the incision was much too large, and the next one would want it half-again bigger. Naka tends to be the most prescriptive," he went on. "He might execute a particular stitch back-hand back-hand back-hand back-hand, and I would do it back-hand fore-hand back-hand fore-hand, and he would tell me it was wrong, although it's just as good. You really learn five different styles of surgery here," he said, referring to the five adult cardiac attendings—Smith, Oz, Argenziano, Stewart, and Naka. "But then it's your job to find the 'sixth style,' the one that is your own."

Argenziano defended the five-style training approach. "When I was a resident," he said, "and I was assisting Craig, I would try to become Craig, and do everything exactly the way he did. Then when I was assisting Mehmet, I would try to become Mehmet. I didn't know whether the differences were just random or had been adapted to some special situation. I've got my own style now, but it still happens that I'll run into some new problem and realize that, oh, the way Craig, or Eric, or Mehmet did this would work well here. And I think it's made me a better surgeon."

The five-style approach also reflects Smith's approach to

division management. It is common for heart surgery departments to take on the personality and operating style of the chief, while the other surgeons become satellites of the divisional star. But the cardiac surgeons at Columbia-Presbyterian are *all* stars, and are widely recognized as such. Mehmet Oz, for example, who is also a prolific author and television personality, is much more widely known than Smith. But Smith argues that multiple styles promote better surgery. "A major program," he said, "brings in a star chief—a 'my way or the highway' guy—in, say, 1991, and he makes it a showplace of 1991-vintage heart surgery. You look at it ten years later, and he's still there, and it's *still* a showplace of 1991-vintage heart surgery. You see it all the time." Sherwin Nuland, the Yale surgeon, made much the same point. "I did advanced training in England in the 1960s," he said, "and they were doing everything differently from how I'd been taught. I thought, Oh, that's terrible, they must be getting awful results. But, of course, they were exactly the same." He went on: "I learned a way to close a belly with just one big stitch, instead of all the meticulous little stitches we use here. But for fifteen years after I came back, I did it the American way. Then I finally decided to do it the way I had learned in England. Nobody objected, and others started gradually to pick it up. If you just have one protocol, you get inbred."

Teaching styles differ even more than surgical styles. Rose, who maintained an active operating schedule even after he became departmental chairman, was known as an unusually gifted teacher. "When I was a resident," Argenziano says, "I'd be doing some procedure, and Eric would suddenly say, 'Turn your back to the anesthesiologist and point your needle holder at the patient's foot.' And I'd laugh, and say, 'what are you talking about?' And he'd say, 'Just *do* it.' So I'd turn my back just as he said, and amazingly, I could move my elbow more freely, or my hands would be better positioned." Oz made a similar comment. "Eric has a great ability to articulate exactly what you're doing wrong. He might say, 'You're doing a backhand stitch at thirty-five degrees, try a fronthand at a hundred thirty-five,' and he'd be right!" Both Oz and Argenziano said they tried to capture some of Rose's granularity in their own teaching—Allan Stewart, only a year out of his residency, remarked to me what a fine teacher Oz had been.

Smith ranks himself as a decidedly *un*gifted teacher. 'Most of what I do is so second-nature," he said, "that I have trouble stepping back and trying to break it into smaller steps." I mentioned that to Oz, who smiled and said, "Eric was like Larry Bird. Craig is Michael Jordan. You wouldn't ask Michael Jordan how he shoots a free throw." Argenziano told me that when you worked with Smith you learned by "osmosis"—which is partly why he had adopted the strategy of trying to become whomever he was assisting. The residents I spoke to greatly admire Smith—Garrido calls both him and Oz "technical geniuses"—but I think all regard him as difficult to assist.

The Worm's-Eye View

All new cardiothoracic residents are stars when they arrive at Columbia-Presbyterian. Columbia tends to see the top applicants in each year's pool—most years, in fact, they see all the applicants. In the couple of resident-selection sessions I sat in on, the surgeons were clearly targeting the very top candidates and have a track record of getting their first choices.

The typical cardiothoracic resident arrives having completed a five-year training program in general surgery, usually with an additional year or two of cardiac-related research—which, if it was at Columbia, would have included taking turns on harvest runs. Most would have served as their general surgery department's chief resident, which is tantamount to a designation as the top resident in that year's class. In general surgery programs, moreover, the requirement that a senior surgeon "attend" every operation is often a thinly disguised fiction, so new cardio-thoracic trainees are already accustomed to operating as independent surgeons. Further, since they risked listing Columbia as their top choice, they clearly regard them-selves as the best of the best, and have seen their exalted self-assessments resoundingly confirmed by residency selection committees.* Cardiac trainees, in short, are not known for fragile egos.

---

*The final placements are determined by a national algorithmic-based system that makes a best-fit match between applicants' rankings of schools and vice versa. The algorithm rewards realism, so both appli-cants and schools are punished for overreaching. That is a classic game-theory paradigm—it's safer to aim low to ensure you get some-thing, because if you reach too high, you might get nothing at all. The same rules apply to the schools. If they pick only top candidates, and those candidates pick a different school, they may not get anyone. It made for extremely intense selection meetings. The selection cycle I witnessed was targeted at a future class, and Columbia once again got its first choices.

But cardiac usually humbles them. "You won't get a good picture of the program from a resident in his first six months," Argenziano me. "They're all overwhelmed." Garrido confirmed that his first months in the program were very rough. "In general surgery," he said, "there are usually just a couple of risky steps, and if something goes wrong, you almost always have time to get help. In cardiac, crises come at you very fast, they're very unforgiving, and they can happen at almost any moment. You're always working down in little holes, so it's hard to see, the sewing is much harder, and stitching tolerances are very small, as little as ten millimeters." Allan Stewart said: "When I did my first cardiac rotation in my general surgery residency, I was sure I didn't want to go into cardiac. It was so brutal. The schedules were brutal, the people were nasty, the complications were severe, and the surgery was hard."

When residents first come to Columbia, they are normally assigned to assist Smith, which ensures that the humbling gets under way from the first day. Mike Bowdish is a pleasant, soft-spoken man in his early thirties who was in the first few weeks of his residency when I was starting the research. Bowdish completed his five years of general surgery residency at the University of Southern California–Los Angeles County Medical Center, and also spent two years at USC's Keck School of Medicine doing research in cardiothoracic surgery. He was drawn to Columbia for its cardiothoracic surgery training, largely on the advice of a Keck mentor who was an alumnus of the division. Bowdish completed his American Board of Surgery certification examinations before joining the cardiothoracic division, and he spent several months working in the division's thoracic section before the start of his formal residency, to ease a sudden staffing crisis.

I first met Bowdish when I came into the OR early one morning to learn more about preoperative patient preparation. I didn't know he was the division rookie, and during the hour and half or so it took to set up the case and open the chest, he appeared wholly at ease and in command of the room, like the qualified surgeon he is. So I was surprised to see the self-assurance disappear as soon as Smith arrived and took over the right side of the table. Smith grunted an acknowledgement of Bowdish's presence, briefly inspected the preparatory work, and proceeded with the bypass and the surgery. His communications with Bowdish seemed mostly a matter of pointing to whatever Bowdish was supposed to be doing next. The only sentence I remember started, "When you go to varsity assisting school, you'll learn that . . . "

As I got to know Bowdish better over the next few weeks, he conceded that he was ill at ease when working with Smith, although he was in awe of him as a physician. Part of the strain, he said, was Smith's habit of commenting only on what you do wrong. And he couldn't yet tell for sure when a Smith silence meant that he was doing okay. Bowdish conceded the program was very tough—I had also seen Argenziano ride him hard one day. But he said it wasn't unusually so; the surgery program at USC by comparison was "malignant."

I mentioned to Argenziano that Bowdish seemed to be struggling. "Almost all us did in the first few months," he said. "In the end, I think he will do very well. He's meticulous, responsible, self-effacing, self-critical. These are good qualities in heart surgery. Some people arrive very confident, very aggressive, but maybe not self-critical, and maybe without really good judgment. Internally, you want someone beating himself up over every mistake, but externally, you want somebody who exudes confidence. We usually reinforce the self-criticism at the start, then later build the confidence back."

Bowdish occasionally kept notes on his operations, so I asked him to expand them and share them with me, which he did for the next couple of months.

I excerpt some of them below. He uses a lot of shorthand and technical terms like "Rastelli" and "Hemifontan": those are names of operations that I won't try to explain. The point is that they were new to Bowdish too, so they give a sense of the steepness of the learning challenge. The bracketed insertions are mine, in an attempt to explain just enough of the shorthand and give just enough context so the reader has a general sense of what's going on.

[A few early notes from January and February.]

1/18: 1st solo cannulation. Went well. [Set up a bypass.]

2/22: Did my first aortic valve replacement with Dr. Stewart today. At the end Allan shakes my hand and says . . . "You just lost your virginity, welcome to heart surgery."

[Next case same day is with Smith. Harvesting a mammary artery to use for a bypass, Bowdish damages the artery. Smith works around it and case okay. Smith tells him:] If this doesn't work I'm gonna take your mammary!

2/27: 1st LIMA -> LAD anastomosis. [Does his first bypass graft, from a chest artery (LIMA) to a major left-side coronary artery (LAD).]

[Some March notes.]

3/20: CABG × 6. [Sextuple bypass.] Yes, × 6! . . . Harvested LIMA RIMA alone completely -> CRS [Smith] shows up as finishing RIMA. Started off-pump -> did LIMA -> FRIMA, LIMA -> LAD, FRIMA -> RI [various coronary grafts], . . . Pt. very wet [bleeding]. 8 HR Case! . . . CRS seemed upset entire case, very gruff.

3/21: Aortic cannulation started some bleeding, but cannulation ok. . . . A hematoma developed. Concerned for dissection. Called CRS . . . [who was irritated] but understood my concern. [In fact no injury, but] I was upset as had wanted to have case set up for him completely.

3/22: MVR [valve repair], CABG × 1. Harvested LIMA, good dissection, easy target. . . . Set up entire case. . . . Cannulation uneventful. . . .

3/23: CABG × 3, BIMA, MV repair, ASD, [atrial septal defect]. Long case. BIMA harvest went well, I was pleased. This is my last case w/ CRS this rotation as he is out next week. He showed up as I was cannulating. SVG -> [leg vein harvest] then he took over. LIMA -> OM1, RIMA -> LAD (in situ), SVG -> PDA. I did $^1/_2$ distal PDA and proximal anastomoses [grafts]. I feel I've made much progress in 3 months—only hope CRS thinks so too! Only discussion w/ CRS was that he no longer wants "Accufuser" [a drug infusion kit] on his patients as they leak too much. I agree.

3/24: Mo [Garrido] did some schmoozing to get me this case. We had 7 cases this day and only 3 fellows. MA [Argenziano] told Mo he'd let me sew the heart in and he did! My *FIRST* heart transplant! MA started while I finished CRS 1st case. . . . It was great. I was probably too tired to really appreciate it yet however. . . . I only hope the cardiologist got the X-match correct! It's now 11 P.M. I'm on the subway home. She's not bleeding and the PA pressures are OK.

3/26: My 34th birthday. Yes, on call of course. Did my usual rounds. Painful call -> just like being an intern. [Events:

+ Patient arrests in the ICU.
+ Another ICU patient needs a chest tube insertion.
+ Spends time with a young girl who needs a double lung transplant and is dying.
+ Admits a patient for Argenziano.
+ Spends two hours inserting a chest tube in a hugely obese man at Garrido's request. Next day attending tells him he didn't want the tube.
+ Escorts a visitor from another medical center.

✦   Checks his transplant patient: doing great.]

3/27: 83-yr old woman [valve case]. Stewart offered me the case. Told me it should take 30 mins [to set up]. . . . It was 45 mins but I was completely ready. X-clamp 58″ [i.e., 58 mins on bypass]. . . . Went very well. You learn that an 83-yr old lady is always just one step from death in cardiac surgery -> very fragile tissue. Stewart quote: "Judgment is what you gain from bad experiences."

3/28: [His transplant] looks good—still extubated. [Valve case] from yesterday extubated, stable, moved [out of ICU]. Short operations are key in old people.

3/28: Stewart told me I did a good job last PM on the [valve case]. . . . Margarita has dinner ready + she's so awesome + good to me. [He has somehow found time for a social life. Margarita is in magazine publishing.]

3/30: [Naka criticizes him for being slow on a LIMA harvest.] I said, sir, I'm just being careful. He finally acknowledged that the LIMA was good, and it's ok if it takes long as long as I improve and do a good job. . . . He let me do $1/2$ of two distals and the proximals, which did not bleed. Overall the case went well. . . . We learned of a tx [transplant] to follow when we finished this case, so at the end, I said, "Yoshi, I think I'm doing the ht tx w/ you." He said, "Yes, you are. I get to torture you more, so go eat, rest, and visualize every step of the operation 100 times."

So the heart tx followed. . . . We started at 4:45 pm

and I had the cannulae in by 5:45 pm—the donor team was 20 mins early but it worked fine. Yoshi is the Jedi Master of heart transplantation. I listened to every step. He let me do 90% of the case—he did a small portion of each anastomosis. I felt I got more "goods" out of him than "sighs." Anyway, the case was awesome, and I had an audience of 20 people. I was like, "Who are all our visitors?" I was so focused I don't remember what they said. Although I had had a long day, I felt very good and alert—it's funny—the strenuous nature of task does much to pull you through. When I have a needle holder in my hand, I forget who I'm with and just operate as best I can. Anyway the transplant went great. She dried up quick and I was home about midnight.

3/31: After a short night I returned. My heart tx was doing well. I did another CABG × 6 with Dr. Naka. It went fine and Naka said the LIMA was good. I came home at 7:30 and was struck by the fact I hadn't come home @ that hour in a month. I wondered if this was the time "normal" people go home! It's funny taking the subway home and walking to my little studio, knowing that I'm one of the few people in the world to ever sew a human heart into another individual.

[April notes.]

4/2: [Sunday] Had day off. Got up and ran in "Scotland Run"—10K in Central Park. I did terrible . . . but it was a gorgeous day . . . spent rest of the day w/ Margarita.

4/3: [Starts pediatric rotation.] Yas [Hirata] is the super-fellow from Japan. He's great. He did an AM case with Mosca, a VSD [ventricular septal defect], and I did my first PDA ligation. [Closed a hole that's normal in a fetus but should close after birth.] I was surprised he let me do the case as I had not done one before. Quick case. Kid did well. It's funny how even though the kids are so small, operating on them isn't that different. It looks scary observing, but when operating is no big deal.

4/4: 2 cases. Yas did a Norwood w/ Dr. Chen and I did a beautiful Rastelli with Dr. Q. . . . He made it look easy and the kid is doing well.

4/5: A sweet case w/ Dr. Q. . . . Quite an elegant little operation. Kid extubated in the OR even! Need to do taxes tonight.

4/6: Hemidiaphragm plication with Dr. Mosca. Case went well. Patient had a shunt and subsequent phrenic paresis. No issues.

4/7: Relatively fun case with Dr. Mosca. Yas was out today. Kid had an AV canal defect, which we fixed with a patch and sewed up the cleft. [At the end] the kid was wet. I gave product and it slowed down, avoiding having to reopen and explore her. Mildly stressful. She did well.

4/8: ASD w/ Dr. Chen -> repaired with a pericardial patch. Learned the "ASD mantra" today. Always iden-tify the following both before and after fixing an ASD

-> the SVC, the IVC, the coronary sinus and the tricuspid valve. You should see all both before and after the repair from the RA [right atrium]. If you don't, you sewed something in *incorrectly*! The case went fine.

4/10: Reop. Bidirectional Glenn with Dr. Mosca. . . . Long, difficult prep. Debate between bidirectional Glenn and Hemifontan. Yes, I really know what those are. We ended up doing a PA plasty and a bidirectional Glenn. Case went fine.

4/12: Another reop. Dr. Q. states this was "one of the most difficult cases I have ever done." . . . Q is amazing. He literally chopped the heart in $1/2$ and put it back together—and it worked. We finished about 9 pm. Q closed her very wet but w/ a bit of product it stopped. I did have to put a chest tube in later.

4/14: [Preemies] look like aliens at that age. So intimidating—but with draping and creating surgical field it always seems relatively "normal" despite the size.

[Then emergency with a baby whose] shunt had clotted last pm but survived as large PDA was still patent. We did a sternotomy and went on bypass. The shunt looked ok, but was clearly clotted. So we did an Ao -> PA central shunt. The kid did fine initially, then about 45 mins p/ closing began to drop his O_2 SATs. We reopened the chest in the ICU because Dr. Mosca was concerned that either the pericardium or the sternum was compressing the heart, but it looked ok. So we closed with a [temporary] patch leaving him open. But the kid continued not to do well. I was making arrangements to return him to the OR when he arrested -> Reopened -> Asystole [no heartbeat] -> Died. Cause? Largely unknown! Mosca et al were quite upset. [The ultimate conclusion was that the baby had a rare tendency toward hyper-clotting. The pediatric surgeons see it from time to time but have never pinned it down to a case type.]

4/19: Was able to leave relatively early. Went home and cleaned my apartment and did laundry. It's amazing how much time those things take when you have so little time to yourself, but I got it all cleaned. Margarita came over about 8 pm. We went to [a favorite restaurant]. About 8:30 pm peds cardiology paged me to inform me that they had accepted a donor in Hershey, Pa. So a donor run. Pickup was at 1:15 am. This was painful as I was on ICU Thursday but I wanted to go. Slept about $1^1/_2$ hours—sort of—but was interrupted [by pager updates] 3 times. We arrived at Hershey 2:45 am. Obnoxious RNs and anesthesiologist claimed not to know about the donor harvest!! So the times got pushed back about $1^1/_2$ hours. We cut about 4 am, X-clamped about 4:50 am. We moved quickly, and I dropped off the heart at [Columbia] at 6:20. Had to present at a 7:30 conference.

I also wanted to get a sense of nighttime call duty, so I arranged to tail Bowdish one night in March when he was "on call." I had been observing an evening case that ended about 9 o'clock, got something to eat, and tracked down Bowdish in the OR, where he was closing up after a Smith case. It had been a long one; the case had started about 3 P.M.—the second case of the day for Smith and Bowdish, and it was now about 10:30. Closing up a bypass patient "in the usual manner," as the case reports say, takes about an hour. One of the very last steps is placing the steel sternal sutures and twisting them, one by one in several passes, to ratchet the two halves of the chest back together. This patient was a very large, heavy man, so the sternal suturing took Bowdish and the physician's assistant, Debbie Savarese, more than ten minutes. As Bowdish gave one last twist to the very last suture to ratchet shut the one tiny remaining opening, the suture snapped with a noise like an air rifle. Bowdish shrugged, Savarese giggled, and they began methodically clipping and removing all the sternal sutures to start over. If nothing else, the harsh surgical training routines inculcate a useful stoicism.

When everything was finished, and the floor was piled with bloody table drapings, towels, and absorbent cloths for the biohazard team waiting in the corridor, a half dozen people—Bowdish, Savarese, Bessie Kachulis, the anesthesiologist, the nurses, the ICU orderly—lifted the patient onto a gurney, rearranged his tubes and drips, covered him with blankets, and we headed for the elevator. It was almost midnight. Bowdish needed to change for his call rotation, and he didn't come with us. It is the anesthesiologist, in any case, who oversees settling the patient in the ICU. When the patient was in bed and on monitors, Kachulis reviewed his charts with the nurses, then headed back to the OR. There was one more case that was still wrapping up.

From a brief personal experience in an ICU many years ago, I had an image of ICU nurses as people of amazing energy and diligence. Columbia-Presbyterian's cardiac ICU is quite new, with enough equipment to fire a space rocket, but the nurses are just as I remembered—active, alert, and aware, even at two in the morning. Twice, amid the cacophony of monitor beeps, I heard the soft, unmistakable, sound of a monitor alarm bell, and each time a nurse was at the patient's side in seconds. The cardiac staff tend to be critical of the hospital's floor nurses, but everyone I asked had a high opinion of the nurses in ICU. The emotional demands are as high as the physical ones—few other jobs provide grief counseling as a fringe benefit. All ICU nurses volunteer for the assignment and are clearly a special breed.

Bowdish arrived in the ICU after a break of about twenty minutes, looking refreshed in clean scrubs and a lab coat. He checked his own patient first, then we made the rounds of the others. There is a simple checklist for ICU rounds. In order of importance, they are: Is the patient bleeding? Is anything else acute going on? And how soon can we get the bed? There are twenty beds in the cardiac ICU, and with up to a dozen adult cardiac operations a day, they can be a critical bottleneck. After checking over one elderly man, he told me that they could move him out in the morning. I thought he looked like hell. Bowdish said, "No. Remember, this is an old man. He came into the ICU only yesterday, there's no bleeding, his tubes are already out, he's healing well, he's awake and knows what's going on. For the second day, he's looking great, so there's no reason to keep him in here. Better to get him out and up."

Floor rounds were next, at the "step-down" unit, which is intermediate between the ICU and the regular floor. A medical student–intern was waiting for Bowdish with patient records and the next day's operating schedule. This was getting on toward 2 A.M. I knew Bowdish had been up for a very long time and should have been exhausted, but he didn't look it—in fact, his face lit up when he saw an upcoming early-morning case: "Oh, I *want* that case! I'll need to get to Mo!"* I saw a patient I had met in the OR the day before, stalking up and down the floor in his bathrobe. He is a gregarious, powerful-looking man who had undergone a minimally invasive procedure and was clearly recovering quickly. He knew I was there as a writer, but waved me over to say that he could never sleep in hospitals and wondered if I could help him get out. I laughed, and he said, "Well, I'm just trying every angle."

Two step-down nurses started lobbying Bowdish for an aggressive intervention in an older woman who had been moved from the ICU the day before and who had been having breathing problems and falling blood pressure. We visited the woman, and Bowdish examined her and spoke

---

*New York has adopted rules limiting resident working hours to not more than eighty hours a week. I had seen Eric Rose, in a surgery recruiting talk for medical students, tell them that the new rules would let them lead a normal personal life. (By comparison, eighty hours is only four hours a week shorter than the twelve-hour–seven-day factory work schedules that outraged nineteenth-century labor reformers.) The State, cleverly, enforces the rules through a private contractor that is reimbursed with the fines it collects from violations. Individual hospital violation rates are not published, but total violations have fallen sharply since the law went into effect. My limited sample suggests that almost all residents, regardless of the intent of the hospitals, do their best to circumvent the rules. This is one of the crucial learning periods of their lives, and they don't want to miss anything that might be important. Smith once commented that they might have to make them wear radio tags.

quietly with her for a few minutes—he has a warm bed-side manner. Then he told the nurses that this was a case he knew well from the ICU and that he didn't think the intervention was necessary. The nurses, interestingly, put him through his paces—not overtly challenging him, but explaining their concerns and waiting for him to defend his decision. Bowdish didn't pull rank, but walked them through his reasoning. The clincher was that a breathing pipe was already in the woman's trachea and she was on a monitor, so if there was a respiratory event, they could relieve her in minutes and then consider a more radical solution. That satisfied them, and they seemed pleased that he had listened.

The rest of the unit was very quiet. Except for my rest-lessly pacing friend and the woman with the tracheotomy, everyone seemed to be sleeping, and there was nothing untoward on the monitors. Sometime after 2:30, Bowdish headed off for a nap in a nearby room. I thought of hang-ing around in case something happened, but was exhausted and decided to go home. The next day, Bowdish told me that, rarely for a call, he had nearly four hours of unbroken sleep, and that the lady with the tracheotomy had been much improved in the morning.

Morbidity and Mortality Meetings

Heart surgery is among the most dangerous of medical procedures. Smith's initial patient interviews always include a line that goes, more or less: "There's about a four to five percent chance of a bad outcome. And by bad outcome I mean death, a stroke, kidney failure, or some other very serious event." So heart surgeons have to get used to seeing patients die or suffer serious injury. Argenziano told me that when he was a resident "there was a bad outcome, and I was involved, and I was just crushed by it. But the surgeon, who had three other cases that day, seemed not to be fazed—he was just moving on to the next case. I had to learn it's not that you don't suffer when something goes wrong, or that you don't see the pain in the family's eyes. But you can't lose your composure, because that puts the next patient at risk." Flora Wang may have said it best: you *swallow* the bad outcome and keep going—especially if you have made a mistake, the patient needs you to stay calm and fix it.

But at some point, you and your colleagues have to sort out what happened. Did you apply the right procedure and execute it correctly, and still lose the patient? Or did you misunderstand the problem? Or did you fumble a procedure? That's why there are Morbidity and Mortality meetings, or "M&Ms." They are a standard feature in surgical practices, although not in other branches of medicine.

The cardiothoracic M&Ms are calendared at a monthly early-morning meeting; each one takes about an hour. Over a span of eight months, I sat in on five of them.* Including

---

*Outsiders are rarely allowed in such meetings. Had the question been posed directly, I doubt if I would have been. Smith had introduced me at one of the regular staff meetings, albeit amid the early buzz of people assembling, and by the time of my first M&M, I was already part of the wallpaper. After the doctors were used to seeing me at M&Ms, most would take the time to explain case details, and I almost always met with Smith afterward to review my understanding of what had transpired.

both cardiac and thoracic cases, there were usually seven or eight cases reviewed each time, so while my sample is hardly scientific, it represents a fair slice of the annual M&M agenda. I didn't keep a tally, but the morbidities— an injury or postsurgical complication—always outnumbered the fatalities. Each case was presented by a resident using PowerPoint slides, and always included the case background, the negative outcome and a brief causal analysis, followed by an open discussion.

The very first case presentation I saw was a mortality, a fairly elderly gentleman who had had heart surgery the year before. Besides bad valves and coronary arteries, he had an astounding list of other things wrong with him— cancer, diabetes, 'cerebral events' (strokes or ministrokes), cognitive issues, infections, and much more. The surgery itself had gone as planned, and he had been stabilized and appeared to be recovering when he suddenly died. At that point, Ralph Mosca interrupted the presenter to ask, "How do you spell 'inoperable'—with one *n* or two?" The clear consensus was that this was a case with a very low probability of a successful outcome—one surgeon estimated 10 percent. When pressed on why they had operated, the resident responded, somewhat lamely, that there was a "large and supportive family who really wanted us to try."

I found it puzzling that a resident was defending the case decision, since the attending is the one who makes such calls. Argenziano later told me that all surgical M&Ms worked that way, and that it was good training. It's true that the residents don't have all the case background, he said, but when a discussion got into details, he and other attendings would take over the discussion of their own cases. One of the first things you learned as a general surgery resident, he went on, was that in big services there were usually one or two natural bunglers, and they would never speak up at M&M. You tried your best not to get assigned to their cases.

Most of the adult M&M cases were very fragile people. Many were in their eighties, some in their nineties, and almost all had important comorbidities—diabetes, obesity, renal issues, often cancer. Such cases are now part of the mainstream in cardiac surgery, even as the rate of bad outcomes continues to fall. But for M&M purposes, it makes it hard to pinpoint what went wrong. There was a woman who had long been bedridden, suffering from an extraordinary list of diseases, but who had made an amazing recovery from a difficult surgery. She became ambulatory again—a great success—then dropped dead while walking on the unit. The family refused an autopsy, so "pulmonary embolisms"—"the ubiquitous PEs," one surgeon said—became the default cause of death. It's plausible: long-dormant detritus in her lungs could have been stirred up by such unusual activity, causing a cerebral or cardiac event. No one really knew.

Frail people are also much more vulnerable to iatrogenic injuries—injuries that medical professionals cause. If you're probing with a metal instrument amid a web of paper-thin blood vessels, you need to be *very* careful. Of the cases I saw, a significant minority seemed iatrogenic, although the evidence was often frustratingly ambiguous. A very ill older woman, for example, had died for no apparent reason shortly after a procedure. The team thought they may have "clipped" her pericardium during a tube insertion; the pathologists couldn't rule it out, but hadn't found clear signs of it.

In another case, an elderly woman had suffered a liver shock during a minimally invasive (small opening) valve repair. The procedure calls for placing a suture in the heart and pulling it slightly toward the surgical opening before placing the aortic bypass cannula. The presenting resident had done the case setup and thought that the shock had resulted from his tugging too hard on the suture. The room was openly skeptical, since he hadn't moved the heart by an unusual amount, but the resident argued that a too-hard pull on the suture could have disturbed the hepatic (liver) artery and stressed the liver. I thought the doctors still looked unconvinced—the resident had a reputation for conscientiousness—and the discussion moved on to the advisability of minimally invasive procedures in very frag-ile patients. (This woman had insisted on it for cosmetic reasons.) Later, I asked Smith his views—he was consis-tently the hardest interlocutor at the M&Ms. His guess was that the resident was right—"He's experienced in that procedure. When he pulled the suture, he must have felt something different to make it stick in his mind like that."

The clearest iatrogenic injury I saw involved another frail, elderly lady undergoing a complex lung procedure. When clamping an artery, the surgeon applied an inappro-priate clamp, an evil-looking tool with toothed, almost scissorlike edges (it was passed around at the meeting). It was designed for clamping tough, thick vessels, not the kind of artery this lady had. The surgeon took the discus-sion himself, but said the nurse had handed him the wrong clamp. Smith picked on that point and pressed the surgeon until he stated that he had not looked at the clamp. For me, it was a fascinating example of the team's ethic at work. Within the group, you declare your errors. I saw it again when a resident recounted how he had inflicted a life-threatening injury during a chest-opening. Although he must have been deeply chagrined by the incident, his presentation was as detailed and deadpan as if he were talking about a case from a textbook. As Mehmet Oz told me, "We all make mistakes. It's part of surgery. The important thing is to be up front about it. Only dishonesty is unforgivable."

The pediatric cases have a flavor all their own. Congenital problems are the mainstay of the practice. Although the caseload is smaller, it comes in extraordinary variety, so procedures are not nearly as standardized as with adults, nor are complications as predictable. Very young children, moreover, frequently react differently from adults, and the variability increases because so many cases come with underlying chromosomal issues. Children with Down's syndrome can be especially challenging: they often present with severe cardiac defects, and it's hard to know how any particular case will react to surgery. Yas Hirata told me that even "normal little kids' circulatory systems are a lot different from ours."

I thought Hirata much the best M&M presenter. His case reports were always meticulously organized and usually included a summary of current research as well as recommendations for future practice. One of his cases underscored the special perils of surgery with little children. Postbypass protocols call for attaching a temporary exterior pacing wire to the heart with a small suture before closing the chest. In most cases, the wire is later removed just by pulling it out, which may cause a momentary pain and a small amount of bleeding. (If a patient has bleeding issues, the wire can be clipped off and left in the chest.) Hirata reported a case in which, after he had removed a wire in the normal way, the child began to cry, then as he became more agitated, hyperventilated and went into cardiac arrest. Hirata responded immediately and the child was okay. His literature search, however, turned up other cases in which little children who got very upset during the postoperative period tipped themselves into arrest. (Absent immediate intervention, cardiac arrest is almost always fatal.) Argenziano recalled one at Columbia. The numbers were small, but scary, and there weren't enough cases to suggest any course of action. Should you warn parents that their child might die if he becomes upset? Argenziano asked. There was not much to do except plant a red flag.

I FOUND the M&Ms very impressive if deeply unsatifying. Within their own frame of reference, they were yet another example of the surgeons' flat, factual, way of dealing with the world. Bad things happen. These are the bad things that happened on our last watch. Some of them were beyond our control. Some others we don't understand. But *these* we could have and should have prevented.

The conclusions they reached were as varied as the incidents. Occasionally, there would be a decision to stan-

dardize a procedure—when to extubate, for instance—
and a working group would be assigned to create a protocol. Occasionally, an incident would trigger an
impromptu study—let's step back, pull the last year's cases
and see if we can discern a pattern. Or someone would
raise larger practice issues: "We've got to pay more attention to the medicine"—meaning being more alert to intestinal or other noncardiac complications. Or: "Are we
withdrawing support too early?"

Most often, however, the lessons were left to be
absorbed into the substrate of personal lore that guides
each of the surgeons' practices. That is the way the old
violin maker's shops worked: "We've tried that new maple
for our backplates. It's not bad, but we need to season it
longer." The overlay of science in heart surgery, of course,
is much deeper than in instrument-making. There is an
immense amount of literature on the circulating debris
dredged up by a heart-lung bypass machine for instance.
But the science doesn't quite take you to the microlevel: is
this patient a good candidate for an off-pump operation
with *this* surgeon? The cardiac M&Ms, like all clinical
training, start with those particularities, but then try to
surround them with principles. Those were the moments
at the M&Ms when the surgeons were most engaged: can
we find a rule here?

Even as clinical exercises, however, the M&Ms have
obvious deficiencies. Sherwin Nuland grumbles that, at
least in larger general surgery shops, they have become
"social-political extravaganzas," demonstrations of "the
art of elusiveness." He fingers the practice of resident pre-

sentations as a central problem, since they often first see a patient in the OR and know little of the actual background of the decision-making. "You would sit there with your mouth dropping sometimes," Nuland said, at the misinformation in a case report. That didn't seem to be a problem at Columbia-Presbyterian, however—at least at the M&Ms I saw—since the responsible attendings almost always took over the detailed analyses of their own cases.

But from a broader perspective, in their role as the primary quality control tool, M&Ms seem quite inadequate. For one thing, they are almost completely unsystematic. The reviews are honest, and within the limits of the forum, reasonably thorough. But there is no database of outcomes and recommendations, no full-time "errors team" cataloging mistakes, seeking out patterns, and recommending changes. And they're incomplete. At the M&M on the Erika Maynard case, for instance, there was no mention of the medication error the week before her death. To be fair, it happened when case responsibility had mostly shifted back to the medical side. I have no idea whether it was relevant, but I'm pretty sure that no one at the meeting knew about it. An M&M without the entire care team, in short, is considerably less than a full examination—but that's how the system is set up. Even on the narrow view that M&Ms should focus solely on surgery, they're still incomplete, since the anesthesiologists aren't there.

Finally, since M&Ms are clinical exercises rather than management forums, they don't even touch huge procedural swathes that have nothing to do with surgical artistry, but can still greatly affect surgical outcomes.

Managing Quality

I enjoy running numbers, and Smith readily gave me access to the division's internal outcome datas. The CABG is a mature procedure with large volumes, so it lends itself to trend analysis. When I graphed the fifteen-year trend line numbers on a spreadsheet, it showed that, in the early 1990s, divisionwide mortality rates were generally over 3 percent, and that they began to drop steadily about 1995. (That is a nationwide phenomenon. The most likely explanation is that the late-1980s expansion of the patient base to include older, sicker patients boosted mortality rates until surgeons developed experience in managing them.) After 1995, the division mortality outcomes are almost always below 2 percent, and Smith has several years below 1 percent.

Except for 2001. On a graph, the sharp upward spike in that one year stands out like an obelisk in a desert. The CABG mortality outcome is about double the average of the previous years, virtually across the division—in effect, all the way back up to early 1990 levels. These were essentially the same doctors, same caseload, same procedures, as in previous years. But since the spike is more than two standard deviations from their trend line, it's highly unlikely that it happened by chance.*

Smith had no problem talking about it. He said that the entire division took alarm as the year went on, and the

---

*The numbers are also reflected in the State outcomes tracking system, an innovation in which New York has led the nation. See Appendix II for a brief description and the Columbia-Presbyterian rankings.

numbers stayed at a high level with no apparent reason—there was even "some paranoid speculation that someone was sabotaging our record." Characteristically, Smith went into an all-court press. He created four-person teams—a surgeon, an anesthesiologist, a perfusionist, and a nurse—to review every mortality, all looking at cases that they hadn't been involved in. They assembled the entire record for each case. The records are almost all paper, and voluminous, but are a rich source of data for professionals taking an in-depth look at a relatively small number of cases. The analyst teams tried to unpack every procedure and pinpoint each step, and they identified more than two dozen procedural changes since the previous year. One of the surgeons, Niloo Edwards, who is now chairman of the cardiothoracic service at the University of Wisconsin, was a devotee of "root-cause" analysis, which is widely used in industry. In effect, you walk the cat back through each branch point in a process, building a retrospective decision tree to pick out turns in the road where something may have gone awry. I read the finished report. It is impressive—both thorough and creative. And it comes up with nothing at all. It led to a few procedural changes, Smith said, but nothing fundamental—and they still had no clue to what had gone wrong. And then the numbers dropped back down to their normal range and have stayed there since.

That is an unsettling experience. For one thing, it reinforces the position of process skeptics like Nuland. The variations among superficially similar patients, many would maintain, compound with the microvariations in apparently identical surgical procedures to produce an uncomputable degree of complexity. Factors like the quality of a blood vessel, the chemistry of the blood, blood pressures, renal balances, lung function, all interact with the elapsed time of the surgery, types of suture, timing variations in medication, how much an organ was handled. No two procedures are ever the same.

But we still have to try. In July, I interviewed Dr. Steven Corwin, the president of New York–Presbyterian Hospital, and a Columbia cardiologist. We spent much of the time talking about medical errors, one of his priorities. He's introduced specific quality objectives for the major departments and has brought in a consulting team from GE to train staff in the famous GE Six Sigma* quality methods. One of the initiatives is a new Medical Event Reporting System (MERS) that is designed around root-cause analytic processes. Any medical personnel can access a MERS Web site and make an anonymous report of an untoward incident. Errors that did *not* result in a bad outcome—"near-misses"—are given the same importance as errors that did.

I'm inclined to give high marks to Corwin and the management team, for New York–Presbyterian (to refer to the hospital, as distinguished from the medical schools)

---

*Six Sigma is statistical shorthand for an error rate of one in less than 3.4 million (or 99.9997 percent accuracy). It evolved originally from high-tech manufacturing process control. Since there are thousands of processes in making a memory chip, they all must be managed to something like Six Sigma levels to produce final yields of 90 percent or so. Nothing that happens in a hospital is controlled at anywhere near that level of accuracy. But even at GE the concept is often employed more as a useful slogan (in financial services operations, for instance) than as a real-world standard.

is consistently ranked among the best American hospitals. A local magazine that has long ranked New York City hospitals chose New York–Presbyterian as number one by a very large margin in 2006. Among ten treatment clusters, the hospital was ranked first in five categories and was second or third in all the others. The largest-margin first-place ranking was in cardiac services, which included cardiology. The magazine lumped the doctors from both the Columbia and the Weill-Cornell medical schools, since they both staff the hospital. And the front-line staff, wherever I've been in the hospital, consistently strike me as unusually courteous and responsive. The attack on medical errors appears to be off to a slow start. Nurses do use MERS and a lot of data are accumulating. Doctors don't use it, however, and there have been only a limited number of root-cause analyses. And although everybody has heard of Six Sigma, few people on the floor seem to know what it is. It's much too early for a fair assessment, however. Corwin's initiatives were still in their first year when we spoke, and hospitals present far more complex management challenges than factories or banks do.

But all hospitals, New York–Presbyterian included, could do a much better job in safety engineering. An anesthesiologist pointed out his OR medication supplies—some twenty identical little clear plastic bottles with small-print labels lined up just behind the operating table. "Couldn't they be color-coded or something?" he asked. "Can you imagine how easy it is to take the wrong one?" And how easy it was for the night nurse in Erika Maynard's case to confuse two of them as she arranged a tray of identical containers in the small hours of the morning. Four or five times—which is far, far too often—I saw a surgeon or an anesthesiologist ask for an instrument or a device, and someone had to leave the OR and hunt it down. On one occasion, a team discovered that a critical machine had been replaced with a new model that none of them had seen before. Johanna Schwarzenberger, an anesthesiologist who trained in Germany, told me that such things were unheard of in German hospitals. Nuland, who also worked in Europe, agreed with Schwarzenberger. In America, he said, you always have the problem of "Sam Stein taking your favorite clamp," but he warned that the spit-and-polish methods of Europe fostered a much more rigid approach to surgery.

Human-factors research—the kind of analyses that focus on precisely such problems—is just now gaining advocates in medicine. A British pediatric cardiac surgeon, Dr. Marc DeLeval, has been applying human-factors methods to the arterial switch, one of the most virtuosic of heart operations. Taking a cue from the airline industry, DeLeval is concentrating on the minor, preventable incidents, such as mistakes in team communications, or "pin-cushioning" (multiple needle pricks to insert anesthesia lines). Airline-based research suggests that it may be the minor complications that are the royal road to catastrophe. That is consistent with what I saw at M&Ms, for few cases could be definitely pinpointed to a major event, like accidently dissecting an artery. It may actually be the accretion of little mishaps that don't show up in the case record that are at fault, if only because they distract the surgeon. Airline "vigilance studies," moreover—epitomized by keeping air traffic controllers alert when all is routine—may be directly appurtenant to anesthesiologists and nurses.

But it would be unrealistic to expect that business quality methods could migrate easily into surgery. Conceivably, we could record every surgical micromotion with multiple digital cameras and construct statistically valid best-practice method books. Would that promote better surgery? I have no idea. It might leave surgeons less able to react to unpredictable events, or slow the development of new techniques. About all that can be said for sure is that the road to modern quality systems will be a long one, and anyone who claims to know the answers probably doesn't understand the problem.*

For the foreseeable future, the best guarantee of surgical quality is likely to remain the artisanal value system itself. When cardiologists, cardiac surgeons, anesthesiologists, and other professionals plan and execute an intervention, they are acting in accord with internalized systems of ethics and the expectations of other professionals. Institutional allegiances or hospital management objectives hardly enter into it. For all its deficiencies, the M&M is a method of quality review adapted to the rules doctors really live by. Medical practice is changing very fast, technology content is soaring, and traditional con-

---

*And may be impossible within the current lotterylike system of redress through tort suit. Accessible and standardized error documentation—who can believe it won't be leaked?—could feed endless lawsuits. Some kind of workman's compensation–type arrangement with expert reviews and an appeal process may be a prerequisite to a completely transparent quality control and fault correction regime.

trol systems have almost certainly not kept pace. New approaches are clearly needed, but they will have to be introduced with care, and it will be the work of many, many years.

But there is another side to the quality challenge. How do you know what works in the first place? Shortly after I came to Columbia, I encountered a tangled tale that is still unraveling as of March 2007. And it suggests what a gnarly question that is.

Chapter 7

THE MEASUREMENT PROBLEM

ON THURSDAY MORNINGS, HEART SURGERY AT Columbia-Presbyterian gets off to a late start to allow time for internal meetings. There are a half dozen or so under way by 6:30—on research projects and the like—and a full staff meeting at 7:30. One Thursday a month, the staff meeting is devoted to "Journal Club," in which four or five recent journal articles are selected for formal presentations by residents. Those were my favorite meetings. Everything a resident does is grist for his final evaluation, so the presentations are usually well prepared, and the surgeons, who are utterly immersed in their craft, become intensely engaged in discussions digging into, say, the fluid-dynamics of different-shaped bypasses.

At one of the first Journal Clubs I attended, in February 2006, the agenda included a recent *New England Journal of Medicine* article suggesting that an antibleeding drug, aprotinin, which is often used in heart surgery, was associated with a number of dangerous side effects, including strokes, cardiac and renal (kidney) effects, and increased mortality. The conclusion was not based on clinical trials, but rather on a statistical analysis of a very large database of surgeries. Since there appeared to be alternative drugs with much the same beneficial effects, the article suggested that continued routine use of aprotinin was "not prudent." The presentation was delivered in a monotone, I was still adjusting to the peculiarities of time in a surgical universe, and this was my second meeting of the morning. Sitting in the back of the room, I mostly concentrated on not visibly drifting off.

Then the resident finished—and to my astonishment, the room almost exploded with anger. Jack Shanewise, the cardiothoracic anesthesiology chief, called the article "completely irresponsible,"and went on that the *NEJM* had been "burned on Vioxx" and was now trying to seize the high ground on aprotinin. (The *NEJM* had indeed published a company-sponsored paper on Vioxx, a blockbuster arthritis drug, that it later discovered had excluded crucial data on cardiac side effects.) All the doctors were seething over the "not prudent" tagline which, I belatedly realized, was doctor-speak for "should be sued." For emphasis, the *NEJM* editors had also included the "not prudent" phrase in its abstract, so it had been widely picked up in the press. The resident flicked back through his PowerPoint slides to a Google search page showing the *New York Times* report on the *NEJM* article. Sure enough, it was bordered by a string of lawyer ads, soliciting aprotinin cases. An older doctor near me murmured, "What kind of a country are we living in?"

Smith focused on the article's methodology: "If you believe in the religion of propensity scoring," he said, "you have to stop using aprotinin. But if you don't have a Ph.D. in math, it's impossible to know whether this is a good study or not." "Propensity scoring" was the primary analytic technique that the *NEJM* study relied on. It is of quite recent vintage, and can retrospectively create simulated clinical trial–style experimental and control groups from large databases. It requires great facility in advanced statistics, large amounts of computer power, and a fair degree of judgment-based data manipulation. And Smith was certainly right that hardly anyone in the room had the mathematical background to judge the quality of the study.*

The discussion went on for almost an hour, and it gradually became clear how deep the doctors' anger was, and how various its targets. Partly, it was simple embarrassment. More than a decade ago, the surgeons at Columbia had developed the first widely used protocols for the safe use of aprotinin. Shanewise arrived much later, but came from Emory University, where the cardiothoracic anesthesiology program is a strong aprotinin advocate. In the year and a half he had been at Columbia, he had been working to *increase* the use of aprotinin. Now here is the *NEJM* telling him, in effect, that he has been "imprudent."

And there was anger over their apparent loss of control over professional standards. Statisticians were now going to tell the surgeons what good medicine was. Almost

---

*Another much-less-publicized study using similar methods was published at about the same time. In comparison with the alternative drugs, it found adverse renal effects related to aprotinin, but not cardiac or cerebral effects, and did not show mortality differences.

everyone in the room felt strongly that in cases where postoperative bleeding was a serious risk, aprotinin had proved to be a highly effective counteragent. But it was not just a matter of opinion. One of the surgeons said, "We've learned not to trust anecdotal evidence. We've had it drummed into us that the gold standard for evidence is the randomized clinical trial." Aprotinin, in fact, had been one of the most studied of surgical drugs. More than sixty randomized clinical trials (RCTs) had almost uniformly demonstrated its safety and effectiveness. While some of the earliest studies suggested the possibility of renal and cardiac complications, they mostly dated from before the Columbia protocols had been widely adopted. Two very large recent "meta-analyses"—studies that combined the results of multiple smaller studies—had strongly confirmed aprotinin's usefulness and safety. But the *NEJM* article dismissed that evidence. Each of the individual studies was small—"underpowered" in the jargon—and apt to miss subtle variations in outcomes. Worse, they were all financed by aprotinin's maker, Bayer, the German pharmaceutical giant.

And the surgeons were angry at the government. Smith said: "The government made the choice to delegate drug testing to the drug companies. There's no money for independent testing. That's why we're in this position." There was also, of course, anger at the tort lawyers. But surprisingly, perhaps the most intense anger of all was focused on Bayer and the corrupting influence of the drug companies. Shanewise said: "There's no one in this room who isn't compromised. You can't go to an anesthesiology conference that isn't paid for by Bayer. Nobody here can say

that they've never had a meal that was paid for by Bayer."
Then he said, "The other night I was attending at an operation on an eighty-five-year-old woman. She was exactly
the kind of case that I think needs aprotinin. And I didn't
know what to do. I finally asked myself, What would I do
if this was my mother on the table—and then I gave her
the aprotinin. Everything came out all right, thank God."

I could sympathize with the surgeons. Old points of reference were visibly wobbling, and the queasiness they felt
was palpable. But I was also pretty sure they were wrong,
and that sooner or later they were going to have to swallow
the study. I had seen the usefulness of "data mining" techniques in business—using powerful computers to discover
unexpected patterns in standard databases—and thought it
was much underused in medicine. At one point in the meeting, Mike Argenziano, who has far more mathematical
training than most surgeons, quietly warned the group that
propensity analyses were producing a lot of useful results
and that they shouldn't dismiss the study too quickly. Later
that day, I walked over to the office of a friend of mine at
Columbia, a senior health care economist, and asked her
to look at the paper. She read it through and said, "I'm not
the one to analyze this in depth, but on the face of it, it
looks like a well-executed study. I'm afraid your surgeon
friends may have to learn to live with it."

It turns out, however, that whatever their reasons for
mistrusting the study, the surgeons' doubts were well
founded. What follows is a twisty tale that is still not completely resolved as of March 2007. But it sheds a stark light
on the challenge of assembling useful medical evidence. The
NEJM study has been, if not quite discredited, strongly

challenged on technical grounds, but some of those same analyses have also helped expose the weaknesses of RCTs. Many RCTs, perhaps even most, are useless or worse. Partly that's because pharmaceutical companies have abused the trial process, but it's also because of the great difficulty and expense of running good trials. Statistical analyses of nonrandomized medical databases, like that in the *NEJM* study, are therefore becoming of crucial importance. But the multiple problems with the *NEJM* paper demonstrate how poorly equipped the medical profession, its professional journals, and its regulators are to take on such a challenge.

The Problem with Drug Companies

The degree of press attention to the *NEJM* article was surprising at first. Although aprotinin creates a nice revenue stream for Bayer—about $300 million in 2005—it has nothing like the public profile of consumer blockbusters like Vioxx or Lipitor, and since it's usually administered on the operating table along with a panoply of other drugs, few patients are even aware of it.

But the alarm over aprotinin came in the midst of a long series of devastating revelations about the ethics and the business practices of "Big Pharma." Movies are usually a good barometer of American attitudes. The central premise of the 2005 hit movie *The Constant Gardener* was that a global drug company was killing poor African children in order to test a highly toxic experimental drug, and commissioning more murders to cover up its crimes. The fact that millions of people apparently found the story perfectly plausible suggests how low the industry's reputation has sunk.

To be fair, the failings of the drug companies are often exaggerated. Drug prices *are* higher in America than in other countries, but by less than usually reported, taking into account the discounts negotiated by managed-care groups and Medicare insurance vendors. In addition, the use of less expensive generics—unbranded copies of popular drugs that have outlived their patent periods—is much higher in America than in other countries, and they are generally cheaper as well. It is also true that drug companies take far too much credit for innovative research—most basic research is financed by the federal government and performed in university laboratories. But there is a large gap between an exciting laboratory compound and a therapeutically useful drug that can be safely absorbed by humans. Creating effective AIDS drugs wasn't as glamorous as decrypting the HIV virus, but was arguably as difficult, and the companies deserve full credit for their achievements.

Still, all accomplishments notwithstanding, the degree of corruption in the drug industry is disheartening. Enormous revenue flows turn on discretionary choices by a variety of gatekeepers—the patent office, the Food and Drug Administration, and, most of all, thousands and thousands of prescribing physicians. Big Pharma's annual lobbying budget, therefore, usually tops that of any other industry, and the companies shower billions of promotional money on working doctors—free drugs, expense-paid trips, lunches, consulting and speaking fees. Getting physicians with financial ties to drug companies off crucial FDA approval committees has been like rooting out roaches. Physicians at Stanford University Medical School were recently advised that they could not be paid for signing journal articles written by drug industry contractors—the mere necessity for such an advisement is itself a comment on the state of some doctors' ethical barometers.

At times, the wrongdoing is not even subtle. TAP Pharmaceuticals, for example, a joint venture between Abbott and the Japanese drug giant Takeda, paid $875 million in 2001 to settle criminal charges and civil liabilities related to its best-selling cancer drug Lupron. (It was overbilling Medicare for the drug in a way that benefited the doctors who prescribed it.) Two years later, AstraZeneca paid $355 million to settle roughly the same charges related to its Lupron competitor. And the year after that, Warner-Lambert, a Pfizer subsidiary, paid $430 million in criminal and civil settlements for illegal marketing of a drug called Neurontin. None of this is *Constant Gardener* territory, but it all lends credibility to the movie's story line.

The *NEJM* aprotinin article therefore fit squarely into an evolving media narrative of scandal at Big Pharma. Bayer charges well over $1,000 a dose for the drug in the United States, which must be fifty to a hundred times its production cost, which it justifies by pointing to the large savings and reduced transfusions from using aprotinin. But there are alternatives. Aprotinin belongs to a class of agents loosely categorized as "antifibrinolytics."* There are two

---

*Fibrin is an important blood-clotting agent. "Lysis" is a kind of molecular destruction. So "fibrinolytic" drugs attack fibrin and prevent clotting, while "antifibrinolytics" help preserve fibrin, enhance clotting, and reduce bleeding.

other, much cheaper antifibrinolytics, operating via different chemical pathways, that appear to have effects broadly similar to aprotinin's. Almost all of the RCTs that demonstrate the benefits of aprotinin are comparing aprotinin to placebos, not to the other antifibrinolytics. But precisely because the alternatives are so inexpensive, no company has been willing to invest in testing them.

The high prices might also be justifiable if Bayer had invented aprotinin, but the drug has been around since the 1920s. Bayer has marketed an aprotinin product, Trasylol, for a very long time—it was occasionally used for certain pancreatic conditions. The company struck gold in the mid-1980s when a British cardiac anesthesiologist, David Royston, made what he calls the "purely serendipitous" discovery that aprotinin had a powerful antibleeding effect. At least a half dozen other companies around the world make aprotinin, but Bayer is the only one that invested in the clinical trials required to win FDA approval of aprotinin as an antibleeding drug for heart surgery. It is also the only one to produce it in an FDA-approved factory and may also have cornered the market on cow lung, the raw material for aprotinin, which is certified free of "mad cow" disease. Even with those advantages, the low cost of the alternatives means that Bayer still must spend heavily on aprotinin promotion—sponsoring anesthesiology events, contributing to anesthesiologists' research programs, and signing up prominent anesthesiologists as speakers and panelists.

Finally, a striking feature of the *NEJM* article is how readily it dismisses the broad array of RCTs attesting to aprotinin's safety and effectiveness, merely on the grounds of their sponsorship by Bayer. In fact, sophisticated industry observers have long since learned to be skeptical of drug companies bearing trial reports.

The Problem with Randomized Clinical Trials

The worst of Big Pharma's corruptions, perhaps, has been the suborning of the clinical testing process—and allowing it to happen may be the greatest failing of the FDA. Clinical tests financed by drug companies, which are the majority of tests, tend to be far more favorable to the companies than tests financed independently—3.6 times as much, according to a recent large survey—and negative test results have been routinely suppressed. A review of tests involving fluoxetine (Prozac) shows how simple-minded the deceptions can be. When fluoxetine is the experimental drug— the one that is being tested—it's typically given in higher dosages than the control drug, so the game is tilted to a positive outcome. Flip the positions, however—so fluoxetine is the control drug—and the dosages are reversed, once again favoring the experimental. Most acceptance trials, in any case, are just against a placebo, even though there may be much cheaper, equally effective, drugs already on the market. Approvals are almost always accompanied by Phase IV agreements, in which the companies agree to conduct further tests to search for side effects and to measure their product against alternative drugs, but the agreements are routinely ignored, without apparent consequence.

If company cheating were the only problem with RCTs,

however, it might be relatively straightforward to fix. But there are factors inherent even in honest RCTs that often make their results unreliable, or outright wrong. For example, if you want an unambiguous test of a drug's efficacy, you need clean experimental and control groups—people suffering only from the target disease and not undergoing any confounding treatments. Compared to people doctors see in their practices, therefore, RCT subjects tend to be younger, freer of comorbidities, and much less likely to be consuming other drugs. One recent study of trials involving nearly 8,500 cardiac-treatment patients showed that the mortality rate of patients eligible to be in the trials, but not enrolled, was twice as high as for the patients actually enrolled in the trials.*

The "end points," or targeted results, in drug trials, moreover, tend to be very simple. For the aprotinin trials, for example, a common end point was the number of postoperative transfusions. When the experimental drug is being compared only with a placebo, and measured on a very precise end point with a fairly large expected effect, fifty, or even fewer, subjects in each of the control and experimental groups is usually enough for statistical significance. So the companies have become experts at calibrating studies to be just large enough to show the effect they want, but not so large as to reveal less obvious side effects, as the *NEJM* charged was the case with aprotinin.

---

*That is a scary finding, for it suggests that researchers may be exercising unconscious bias in trial patient selection within the pool of those who are officially eligible. Or, conceivably, trial patients get much better care than normal patients, or both selection and treatment factors may be at work.

Meta-analyses, aggregating smaller studies, are often help-ful, but can easily be confounded by relatively minor divergences in the smaller studies.

But the most important problem is that it is so hard, and so expensive, to run good RCTs. The National Insti-tutes of Health (NIH) recently completed a classic study of hypertension drugs, involving four expensive prescription compounds and a traditional generic diuretic. To the experts' surprise, the diuretic came out the clear winner on both effectiveness and safety. One of the prescription drugs was proven so dangerous that it was actually with-drawn. But the study involved 42,000 subjects and took eight years to complete. Another large-scale study is under way in Canada, sponsored by the local NIH equivalent, that should finally resolve the controversy over aprotinin. Commencing in 2002, it involves a comprehensive analy-sis of 4,000 cardiac surgery patients in 600 institutions throughout Canada, and will include aprotinin and both of the alternative drugs. Results should become available starting in 2008.

Trials of surgical techniques or medical devices are even harder to mount than drug trials. Sherwin Nuland, the Yale surgeon and a specialist in medical ethics, maintains that it is "not possible" to run RCTs in surgery. Subterfuges, like making an incision to simulate a surgical intervention, or to implant a dummy device, arguably violate the precept to "do no harm," and few doctors are willing to cooperate in such ruses. Surgical technology is also continuously evolving. Several large trials of heart bypass surgery were implemented over periods when outcomes were rapidly improving, which greatly complicates their interpretation.

In surgical trials, moreover, all comparative analyses are inevitably confounded by variations in individual technical skill—some surgeons would get better results with almost any procedure.

Undertakings like the NIH hypertension study and the Canadian aprotinin study are surely what we have in mind when we talk about RCTs as the "gold standard" for medical evidence—studies with the scale, financing muscle, and analytic firepower to provide definitive answers to important questions. But it is hopelessly infeasible to apply that order of screening to every new therapy in the explosion of invention emanating from our university and company laboratories. The "gold standard" RCT will almost always be more of a platonic than a practical ideal. Insisting that RCTs are the only useful medical evidence merely begets a pestilence of *bad* RCTs that benefit no one but the purveyors of questionable medicine.

So the quest to develop a toolkit of reliable statistical techniques to supplement, or possibly replace, RCTs is an important one, and the "propensity scoring" approach used in the *NEJM* article, is one of the more promising of current candidates.

The Promise of Propensity Scoring

In an ideal world, the oceans of medical records held by hospitals and other providers should be a rich source of information on the safety and effectiveness of medical procedures. But even if records were more accessible to researchers, making effective use of them would be problematic. In the research jargon, they are merely "observational" databases: causal associations derived from them are generally regarded as meaningless. To see why, assume you were trying to analyze the mortality effects of smoking from a large, but uncontrolled, database. A direct comparison of the mortality rates of pipe smokers and cigarette smokers would probably show that cigarette smokers have the better life expectancy, which seems odd, since cigarette smokers are more likely to inhale. The puzzle goes away, however, if you plug smokers' age into the database. Pipe smokers tend to be older than cigarette smokers, and on an age-adjusted basis, cigarette smokers actually do have the higher mortality rate.

A simple way to make the age adjustment is to stratify the sample by age—say, comparing everyone 20–24, 25–29, 30–34, the finer the strata the better—and the age relationship will be readily apparent. In real life, however, any large, interesting set of observations will contain so many "confounding variables"—variables that could affect outcomes of interest—that the subgroupings (pipe smoker, aged 20–24, overweight, and upper income) quickly become unmanageable. Powerful desktop computers now permit analysts to tackle very large data sets with mathematical tools, like "multiple regression analysis," that can often correct for biases buried in the data. While they are very useful, such tools can also be "remarkably misleading," in the words of one expert, primarily because of assumptions embedded in the software about the normal behavior of databases.

Propensity scoring was developed in the mid-1980s to improve the validity of data extracted from observational databases. For example, suppose you have a large observational database of cardiac patients who have been treated either with surgery or only with medication, and you want to study their comparative mortality rates. The problem, of course, is that doctors are strongly disposed to recommend surgery for the sickest patients, so you would expect them to have high mortality rates.

The propensity analyst would approach the problem by first identifying a wide range of variables that might relate to the referral for surgery, like left main disease, multiple occlusions, etc. She would then use standard software to run hundreds or even thousands of multiple regression analyses to tease out which variables are most important, and the strength of each relationship. Each variable's influence on the referral decision would be captured in a propensity score. The separate scores for each variable can then be combined into an overall score for a patient that approximately captures the likelihood of his being referred for surgery.

And now comes the rabbit out of the hat. The analyst can then stratify all the patients in the database by their propensity scores, in the same way as we stratified smokers for age. The patients in each stratum are then more or less equally likely to have been referred for surgery, whether they actually were or not. *But that's not a bad definition of a randomly selected group.* The whole point of random selection is to ensure that people selected in the control group had an equal chance of being in the experimental group, so selection bias is eliminated. The propensity analyst can therefore proceed to analyze each of the matched strata as if it were the output of a real RCT.

That capsule description also suggests the limitations of propensity scoring. In the first place, you can never be sure that you haven't missed an important confounding variable. The clinching advantage of randomized studies is that, as long as the control and experimental groups are large enough, all of the important variables will be more or less equally represented in both groups, whether or not the analyst is aware of them. A second problem is that propensity analysis is not an impersonal, algorithm-driven, processing job, like a multiple regression. Instead, the analyst is constantly making crucial judgment calls—selecting the initial variable set, deciding how deeply to dig for unknown confounding variables, constructing the subgroupings, and many others. Dr. Eugene Blackstone, a heart surgeon who has made a personal mission out of spreading the propensity scoring gospel, says "it takes lots of love" to build a propensity scoring data set, remassaging the data again and again before constructing the final data structure.

Just on its pedigree, the *NEJM* aprotinin study commands attention. The primary author, Dennis Mangano, is both a cardiac anesthesiologist and a mathematics Ph.D., and heads the Ischemia Research and Education Foundation, dedicated to improving the treatment of diseases marked by insufficient arterial perfusion. The foundation does not accept funds from pharmaceutical or medical device companies and has been a pioneer in the application of propensity methods to cardiac research. One of its, and Mangano's, major accomplishments has been the construction of a very large observational database of CABG patients that includes nearly 7,500 data points on more than 5,000 patients drawn from 69 hospitals in 17 countries. The data were collected between 1996 and 2000, and Mangano has used them for several other well-received analyses. A 2002 report, for example, is considered a decisive demonstration of the great value of aspirin therapy after bypass surgery.

The results from the *NEJM* aprotinin study, moreover, were quite stark. Patients receiving aprotinin seemed much more likely to suffer renal failure or require dialysis, and there were also statistically significant increases in death rates, and adverse myocardial and cerebral events. Further, most adverse outcomes in the aprotinin group were dose-dependent—they were much more likely to occur in high-dose patients. And the side effects were much less frequent with the alternative antifibrinolytics. Unusually for a propensity-based study, Mangano also presented a forceful review of clinical and laboratory data supporting his statistical findings. Aprotinin has a strong affinity for the kidneys, and there are reasons to believe that it may damage the renal tubules; other research lent plausibility to its potential myocardial and cerebral effects. Warning signs of kidney damage had long since cropped up in the randomized clinical trials that had supported the drug's safety, and the FDA had specifically cited the the danger of "kidney toxicity" in its original approval letter. But, as Mangano acidly notes, company-sponsored trials were generally too small to kick out an unambiguous conclusion on renal effects.

Mangano concluded by briefly acknowledging the pitfalls of propensity scoring, but maintained that since a large and unusually thorough study had uncovered real dangers associated with aprotinin, and since safe alternatives were readily available, he had made his case. As he put it in a later exchange, "shouldn't we now err on the side of protecting the patient . . . instead of protecting the drug?"

The Problems of Propensity Scoring

Strikingly, after the initial shock of the Mangano release wore off, the anesthesiology profession more or less officially closed ranks in favor of aprotinin. An updated set of surgical "Practice Guidelines" issued by the American Society of Anesthesiologists in July 2006 maintained its previous recommendation regarding the use of aprotinin, pointedly ignoring the Mangano study and citing only the RCT-based meta-analyses on aprotinin's safety and effectiveness.

A reaction against propensity scoring appears to have been brewing for some time. As early as 2000, an *NEJM* editorial worried that the spread of statistical analytic techniques threatened to undermine the commitment to RCTs, which it called the only sure way of eliminating patient selection bias. Propensity scoring, in particular, since it is one of the more accessible of the newer approaches, seems to be popping up in almost every issue of most of the major journals. One recent paper suggests that with the proliferation of the technique, the quality of the studies has been slipping, and many appear to be badly conceived.

I reached out to Donald Rubin, a professor of statistics at Harvard. He is the coinventor of propensity scoring and has written widely on its applications. My email drew an immediate response:

The analyses by Mangano et al. are a misapplication of propensity score methods and should not be the basis of any conclusions regarding the use of aprotinin. I am surprised the study was considered publishable by any journal. My criticisms are numerous.

He also told me, however, that he had been engaged by Bayer to consult on their response to the article, and we agreed I should look for an expert without ties to any of the parties.

The detailed criticisms below are based mostly on discussions with two professional statisticians, Stan Young and Bob Obenchain, both with a substantial record of scholarly publication in statistical methods. Dr. Young was a public witness at a September 2006 FDA hearing on the aprotinin controversy. He is director of bioinformatics at the National Institute of Statistical Sciences, a university-sponsored consortium in North Carolina's Research Triangle, and an adjunct professor of statistics at three universities. Young has no relation with Bayer and was not paid for his time at the hearing; he was there, he said, "solely because I take the misuse of statistics personally." He is also, however, a thirty-year veteran of the industry, and pharmaceutical companies are among the institute's affiliates.* Dr. Obenchain has had a long career at Eli Lilly, where Young was also employed, and is an expert on propensity methods. Finally, Bayer submitted a

---

*The institute's affiliates include thirty universities, ten government agencies, two of which are NIH units, and fifteen large companies, five of which are pharmaceutical companies. Bayer is not one of them.

briefing paper prior to the September hearing with a detailed critique of Mangano's methods, which I assume was partly Rubin's work.

I've extracted three classes of criticisms of the Mangano paper, only one of which is technical. The first relates to evidence of carelessness in the presentation. In scholarly articles, authors also prepare abstracts—short summaries of the article's main points. The abstract for the Mangano article includes the conclusion that "aprotinin was associated with a doubling of the risk of renal failure requiring dialysis among patients undergoing complex coronary-artery surgery (odds ratio 2.59[)]." The "odds ratio" means that the patients given aprotinin were 2.59 times more likely to suffer dialysis-requiring renal failure. That was arguably the most damning charge against aprotinin and the one most widely picked up by the lay press. It was also *not* what the article actually said. If one goes through the tables of data, they show that aprotinin patients undergoing complex heart surgery were 2.59 times more likely to suffer a *renal event*, which was defined as *either* a renal failure requiring dialysis or an increase in serum creatinine levels. An increase in serum creatinine levels is suggestive of renal problems and clearly not a good thing, but it is often transitory, and there are a number of effective treatments, like ACE inhibitors. Lumping catastrophic outcomes like near-total kidney failure together with changes in chemical markers, especially without providing any information on the proportion of each, seems obfuscatory at best. But misstating an important result in the abstract is sloppy in the extreme. That the editors of so prestigious a journal as the *NEJM*, in a piece calculated for maximum impact, would let such a howler slip by is incomprehensible.

Second, the article is full of anomalous details that call for explanation. For example, a large group of database patients with very high death rates were excluded from the analysis. Depending on whether they received aprotinin or not, they could greatly skew the outcomes, but there is no explanation as to why they were excluded. Mangano has also issued several reports based on this same database in the past, but the heart attack death rate is much higher in this report than in any of the previous ones, again with no explanation. Mangano's analysis also appears to omit several potentially important confounding variables. Germany, for example, uses aprotinin far more than any other country, so German patients must be disproportionately represented in the aprotinin group. But Germany also has a very high cardiac mobidity and mortality rate, suggesting that the reported adverse outcomes just confirm the Germanness of the aprotinin group.* Certain treatment variables that are strongly associated with adverse outcomes, like time on bypass and the use of fresh frozen plasma products, also appear to have been excluded. Finally, Mangano states that his methods achieved the magic propensity balance among people receiving and not receiving aprotinin. The article's aprotinin patients, however, were much more likely to have certain risk factors

---

*Conceivably, of course, aprotinin may be the *cause* of the high German morbidity and mortality rates. But practices differ so much from country to country that it would require a substantial research effort to pinpoint the causes of the German variance.

than the other patients, and the disparities are large enough to suggest that it might have been difficult to construct useful subgroups.

While the questions in the preceding paragraph raise flags, and there are a lot of them, Mangano may well have satisfactory answers for them all. Which brings us to the third problem: the secrecy surrounding his data. As of March 2007, more than a year after the publication of his article, Mangano has refused to release his underlying data and detailed analyses. A critical test of scientific claims is that they can be replicated by other workers. The National Academy of Sciences has adopted principles that require authors of scholarly articles to make their data freely available to other researchers. Similarly, FDA approval submissions must contain all relevant data in a form suitable for reanalysis by the agency's statisticians, since it is the only way to be sure that claims are truly supported. But the same considerations apply to Mangano.

Mangano's unwillingness to submit his data seems perverse—there is almost no way that the FDA could overturn a previous approval that was based on a substantial body of statistical material simply on his say-so. Publicly, Mangano insists that he did offer up his data, but that is disingenuous. At a September 2006 public hearing, before a panel of expert FDA advisors, Mangano made it clear that he would allow FDA staff to look at the data, but only on his computer and while he was physically present, and he categorically refused to give them the data so they could analyze it themselves. Negotiations had stretched on for months. As the FDA representative stated at the hearing:

We were offered limited access to the data. There was this qualifying expectation that our examination be chaperoned, or supervised, if you will. . . . Our statisticians felt uncomfortable having a supervised access to that data in the sense that we would not have the ability to explore the data and at least verify the mathematics and the statistical aspects.*

Given that background, it is surprising that an *NEJM* editorial published on November 23, 2006, should state that Mangano had "offered the FDA unrestricted access to the data, but the offer was not accepted." Mangano, indeed, made that claim in a letter that accompanied the editorial, but the *NEJM* editors must have known what had actually transpired. I later corresponded with Dr. William Hiatt, of the FDA's Cardio-Renal Advisory Committee, who chaired the hearing. He told me he hoped the FDA staff would execute a full propensity analysis with the Mangano data, which seems reasonable enough, but that would entail a couple of months of work at least, and would be impossible under the Mangano restrictions.

A second observational study, by a Canadian anesthesiologist, Keyvan Karkouti, was also presented at the hearing. It used classic propensity-matching methods to compare outcomes from aprotinin and tranexamic acid, one of the two cheaper antifibrinolytics in nearly a thousand "moderately high-risk" patients. It was not favorable to aprotinin. Aprotinin was no more effective than

---

*The notes to this chapter include an extended excerpt from the hearing exchanges on this point. See pages 291–295.

the cheaper alternative and had significant renal effects, defined as increased creatinine levels, but no increased mortality, or additional strokes, cardiac, or cerebral events. There were also more cases of renal failure in the aprotinin group, but not at the level of statistical significance. Karkouti clearly laid out his methods and furnished all the supporting data to the FDA. No one, including the Bayer representatives, challenged his findings, and it helped confirm the committee's conviction that aprotinin was associated with renal effects.

At the end of the hearing, left with little choice, the expert panel voted 18 to 0, with one abstention, to ignore the Mangano paper and maintain, with some minor adjustments, the current recommendation supporting the use of aprotinin for patients at a high risk of bleeding. In doing so, they specifically recognized the presence of renal effects, but felt that they were outweighed by the dangers of extensive bleeding in high-risk patients. They were unconvinced that aprotinin caused "renal failure requiring dialysis" since the number of observed events was very small, and they saw no evidence of elevated mortality risks, or cerebral or cardiac events. Finally, they noted that while the effects on aprotinin in reducing transfusion requirements were well established, there were no data to support the assumption that it thereby improved mortality.

Soap Opera

With the advisory committee essentially confirming the value of aprotinin in appropriate cases, the undermining of the Mangano study seemed complete. But *then*, a week after the FDA hearing, Dr. Alexander Walker, a former chairman of the Department of Epidemiology at Harvard University, informed the FDA that he had been engaged by Bayer's German parent to carry out an analysis of aprotinin effects from a claims database maintained by United Healthcare, a large HMO, and apparently had come up with results not unlike Mangano's.

The FDA naturally suspended its review of aprotinin until it could analyze the new Bayer data. While the agency's press release was couched in bland officialese, several of the advisory committee members expressed outrage at Bayer's behavior. Bayer claims it fully intended to release the data once its analysis was completed. In any case, their failure to disclose that they were undertaking such a study was itself a violation of their terms of engagement with the FDA. In the wake of multiple revelations that companies were repressing data unfavorable to their products, the FDA had reconfirmed the requirement that companies fully disclose internal studies on the performance of drugs under agency jurisdiction. The company has "reassigned" the two executives who contracted for the study, and in time-honored corporate damage-control style has engaged an outside counsel to review what went wrong with their internal processes.

Walker's approach is an appealing one. Claims databases are usually regarded as not useful for treatment analyses because of the frequency of coding errors and the incentive to overcode. Walker finesses the problem by inferring disease chracteristics from treatment patterns— the tests, the prescriptions, the number of visits, etc.—

rather than from codes. Assuming his methods withstand critical analysis, they offer a nice counterpoint to Mangano's approach. Mangano's CABG database is highly detailed, and has fed several studies, but was very expensive to construct, and will inevitably obsolesce as treatments evolve. Walker, on the other hand, should be able to quickly extract at least indicative results on a variety of questions, and his results will gain authority from the very large databases he draws from. His aprotinin study reportedly involved more than 60,000 cases and was executed in just a few months.

As of March 2007, the FDA has still not reacted to the Walker study, and Walker himself is under a confidentiality rule. In December 2006, however, the agency released a label update for aprotinin that includes a modest toughening of restrictions, all of them consistent with the consensus of the advisory committee. The most extensive warnings related to the possibility of anaphylactic shock in patients who have had previous exposure to the drug, an issue that was not discussed in Mangano's *NEJM* paper. (Anaphylaxis is an immune response; it occasionally causes a fatal reaction to bee stings in sensitized individuals.) The new label also added an explicit warning on the risk of renal dysfunction but noted that such effects were most common in people with preexisting renal conditions, and usually were "not severe and [were] reversible." Finally, it reinforced the use indication by adding, in italics, that aprotinin should be restricted to patients *"who are at increased risk for blood loss and blood transfusion."* There was no mention of Mangano's paper, and the cited evidence was all drawn from meta-analyses of accumulated RCTs. (FDA drug labels, it should be noted, are quasi-advisory. Doctors may legally prescribe an approved drug for anything at all, although companies are barred from marketing off-label uses. Off-label applications for aprotinin in fields like orthopedic surgery outstrip on-label use.)

While Mangano and the *NEJM* deserve credit for precipitating both the label review and a rethinking of the trend toward increased aprotinin use, their primary findings on mortality risk were clearly rejected by both the FDA and the anesthesiology profession, and the episode has probably raised the barrier to professional acceptance of statistical results from observational databases. The FDA's silence on the Walker study is perhaps to be expected. Given the novelty of his methods, the likely next step would be to convene an advisory committee meeting to review his methods and conclusions, probably in the summer of 2007. Our story, therefore, ends on an inconclusive note—a tawdry melodrama still missing parts of the final act.

But since we're on the subject of soap opera, an earlier act in the play still puzzles: what on earth was going on at the *NEJM*?* Poking a powerful profession in the eye, as the Mangano article did, is part of a journal's job. But the most lethal mode of scholarly assault is usually to downplay the rhetoric and let the data speak for themselves. In this case, the presentation was oddly tilted almost to pro-

---

*An *NEJM* spokesperson told me that they never give interviews on editorial decisions. I also made several requests to Mangano for interviews, and sent him written questions, but he did not reply.

voke a fight. The article's tone was often caustic, doctors complained that press releases went out well before the article was available, and there was the stark "not prudent" conclusion highlighted in the abstract. Nothing wrong with that, *if* your data are unassailable. But the paper is so shot through with apparent inconsistencies that the professional associations and the FDA have effectively ignored it.

A little history, however, suggests that the *NEJM* may have been anxious for a confrontation. The current editor, Jeffrey Drazen, was appointed in 2000, succeeding two crusading editors, Marcia Angell and Jerome Kassirer, who are strong critics of the drug industry. Since their departures, both have published exposés of medical corruption in general and the pharmaceutical industry in particular. The choice of Drazen was especially controversial, for he had had financial relations with twenty-one pharmaceutical companies between 1994 and 2000, the half dozen years before his appointment. Early in his tenure, the *NEJM* published the flagship study that established Vioxx as a multibillion-dollar product—the now-famous paper that withheld the data on cardiac events that later led to the drug's withdrawal. As those cardiac data became known, the *NEJM* published an expression of concern about its earlier paper in December 2005, and after allowing the authors a chance to explain themselves, withdrew the article in March 2006. A few weeks later, however, the *Wall Street Journal* revealed that the *NEJM* had been informed of the data discrepancies by a knowledgeable third party as early as 2001. Criticism of Drazen and the *NEJM*, especially in the British medical journals, was vitriolic—the episode was more proof "that medical journals are an extension of the marketing arm of pharmaceutical companies," as the *Journal of the Royal Society of Medicine* put it.

The Mangano study would have been in preparation for publication at about the same time the embarrassing revelations on Vioxx were being broadly released. Drazen and the other *NEJM* editors knew that they would be fiercely criticized. What better way to prove their *cojones* than to go full-bore against aprotinin? The *NEJM*, after all, is also a big business with estimated profits of perhaps $75 million a year. An impression that the journal, or its editor, is an industry patsy may not be good for sales. Dennis Mangano, with his antiestablishment reputation is the perfect antidote, and he has done good work in the past. But that is no excuse for suspending standards.

This is a sad, messy tale. But perhaps some good may come of it. New devices, new procedures, and new medications are proliferating at an accelerating rate, and it is simply not possible to subject them all to "gold standard" RCTs. So enthusiasm for the statistical treasures potentially lurking in medicine's vast observational databases is entirely justified. And by assembling his database of heart surgery patients Mangano has done a signally important piece of work. But as frequently happens in the early stage of a hot new procedure, enthusiasm can overweigh judgment. Journals should simply stop publishing statistics-based claims from observational data—like each month's boatload of new articles based on propensity scoring—until they have assembled panels of expert reviewers, just as they do for medical claims. (And doctors who have had a couple of courses in statistics are not experts.) Upgrading capabilities for handling advanced quantitative methodologies will not be a trivial undertaking for medical journals, and may require substantial reworking of current acceptance processes. But if they are not prepared to make those investments, they should stay out of the game.

As soap operas go, and this one has been especially depressing, it could still have a happy ending. One of the FDA advisory panel members, David DeMets, chairman of the biostatistics department at the University of Wisconsin, said in his closing remarks:

> Well, this has been a fascinating day. . . . [W]hen I looked at the *New England Journal* paper I was disturbed by it. . . . I pretty much dismissed the conclusions that were drawn. But . . . the reason it's been fascinating today is. . . . [i]n the post-Vioxx era . . . we're going to have to rely on observational data of this kind to make, to get, some further information. We will not have randomized trials of long duration for rare events. But I think today's discussion has demonstrated just how big a challenge that is. . . . It's very tricky stuff and it's very hard to do. . . . We're going to have to really drill down on the analysis details a lot more than we do in, say, randomized trials.

I think that's exactly right, and if it results in medical journals upgrading their abilities to handle advanced quantitative arguments as well, that would be a happy ending indeed.

Chapter 8

THE FUTURE OF HEART SUR- GERY

THE ANNUAL TCT, OR TRANSCATHETER CARDIO-
vascular Therapeutics, conferences must be the biggest,
slickest, most spectacular medical gatherings in the world.
The one I attended, the weeklong TCT2006, held at the
cavernous Washington (D.C.) Convention Center in late
October 2006 could boast of 11,000 attendees, most of
them cardiologists, from eighty countries. The main
opening event, held in three large ballrooms with
retractable walls removed, had seating for 3,000, but was
still lined with standees. Two other large opening events
plus multiple smaller ones were in session at the same
time. The multimedia wall display in the main room was
perhaps a hundred feet wide, with a curved black-leather-
and-rosewood conference table stretching thirty or forty
feet along its base.

The founder and guiding spirit of the TCT is Martin
Leon, who was welcoming his guests from the ballroom

podium. He is fifty-five, personable and low-keyed, and one of the most influential interventional cardiologists in the world. Interventional cardiologists thread catheters, or long, thin tubes and wires, through blood vessels to get access to the heart. Using tiny, catheter-based tools and devices, they can perform many tasks, such as reopening an occluded coronary artery, that were once the exclusive domain of open-heart surgeons. Leon, an outstanding practitioner and innovator, is a former director of interventional cardiology at the NIH and founder and chairman of the Cardiovascular Research Foundation. His day job is as associate director of the interventional cardiology program at Columbia-Presbyterian.

After Leon's opening remarks, the wall display dissolved to the catheter lab at Columbia-Presbyterian, where a team headed by his partner and Columbia interventional cardiology director, Jeffrey Moses, was about to perform a difficult procedure on a real patient, using a "rotablator," a miniaturized tunnel-digging machine. As the operation proceeded, multiple windows on the wall display zoomed seamlessly from teamwide shots, to meticulous closeups of the catheter insertion, to images of the catheter threading its way through the arterial system. Windows popped open and closed as shoptalk bounced back and forth between Moses' team and Leon and the twelve other famous cardiologists at the main table—about rotablator rpms, balloon pressures, wire diameters. At one point, when the rotablator got stuck, Leon looked almost happy. "Okay [addressing the audience], this is a great teaching case. You have to realize these are difficult procedures. Now, Jeff, how will you get that out?"*

The rotablator was freed, but the case was far from finished when the Columbia team waved good-bye, and the display wall dissolved to a transatlantic cartoon trajectory to Milan, swirling shots of La Scala and other landmarks, "Grand March" trumpets from *Aida*, then Antonio Colombo and his team at San Raffaele Hospital waving "Hello, Martee." Leon and the other head-table cardiologists kibitzed enthusiastically as Colombo placed a tricky V-shaped stent, or wire-mesh support, in a diseased arterial branch point. But precisely at thirty minutes, the room was teleported away, with a flourish of samba and clips of Carnaval revels, to an operation in São Paulo, and from there, finally, to one in Rotterdam. All the procedures were cutting-edge, all the teams were world-class, and all of them were clearly friends of Leon.

The several days I was there followed that pattern—dozens of events, packed rooms, flawless tech-dazzle. Sponsor banners from drug and device companies festooned the halls, and one large floor was mostly given over to company displays. All of cardiology's industrial giants were there—GE, Siemens, Philips, Medtronic, Toshiba, Cordis, Boston Scientific, Abbot Vascular, Edwards—plus an army of hopefuls, like Bioheart (cell-based heart regeneration), Atritech (a clot catcher), Cardia (tool to close sep-

---

*During a similar display at the 2004 TCT, a procedure went seriously wrong, and the patient died later that day. But Leon has stuck to the same live format. As I'll show later in the chapter, he is seriously committed to showing *everything*. Rather than sugarcoat difficult operations, he stresses the dangers.

tal holes), and many others. The pharaonic assemblies, the parade of companies, the sheen of serious money, all drove home that interventional cardiology is "hot."

And that cardiac surgery is very much on the defensive.

I first met Leon when I sat in on a meeting between him and Craig Smith in early 2006. The meeting was ostensibly an administrative one—finding space to create a "hybrid OR," equipped for both cardiac surgery and interventional cardiology. But it was really about the future of heart surgery.

Interventional cardiology developed more or less side by side with the boom in cardiac surgery starting in the mid-1960s, initially as a diagnostic handmaiden, but as the TCT demonstrated, increasingly as a competitor. The first cardiac catheters were used to measure blood dynamics within the heart, then to pinpoint blockages by squirting dyes through suspect arteries. But cardiologists discovered that they could use the catheter to push aside coronary occlusions, and catheterization became a first-line defense after a heart attack. The next steps were to expand constricted arteries with tiny balloons, then more permanently with metal stents. Catheter-based tools are now progressing very rapidly. At least one company is marketing a micro cardiac pump that can drive a full complement of blood, in effect, a button-sized proto artificial heart on a wire.

The discussion between Smith and Leon was an easy one—Smith is too rational, and Leon too emollient, to imagine it otherwise. They pretty quickly settled on a boundary line between cath lab procedures and those that required a full-blown cardiac surgery OR and staffing. They also agreed, resources permitting, to create two hybrid ORs that would support either cardiac surgery or catheter interventions, and reached a rough consensus on capital requirements. The cardiologists need walls full of catheters and guide wires, and far more elaborate imaging equipment than surgeons use, while the surgeons' open-chest working environments impose the most demanding sterility requirements and a staff quotient tuned to the probability of disaster. (Cardiac cath labs ship their disasters to a surgical OR.)

The hybrid OR was completed just about the time of the TCT conference. The hospital was willing to support only one, not two, and they chose to locate it within the cardiology suite, a not-so-subtle signal of shifting specialty pecking orders. The hybrid OR is ideal for the more invasive cardiological procedures that require surgical-quality sterility and backup, as well as for true hybrid operations —I'll describe an important one later—that incorporate both surgical and catheter-based techniques. The longer-range objective is that a hybrid procedural environment will speed the evolution of a new breed of "cardiac interventionalist" trained in both surgical and interventionalist disciplines. The Columbia surgeons and cardiologists have already established one of the first combined residencies in interventional cardiology and cardiac surgery. Mat Williams, the first joint fellow, who completed his cardiothoracic surgical residency in 2005 and his interventional cardiology training in 2006, now holds a joint appointment as a Columbia-Presbyterian interventional cardiologist *and* cardiothoracic surgeon, with full privileges in both departments, the first such position in the nation.

For a cardiac surgeon, Smith has been unusually open-minded toward the advances of the cardiologists, and seems to have become one of their favorite surgeons—he was one of the few surgeons on a panel at the TCT conference, for instance. His more closed-minded brethren, however, might protest that he has the luxury of an overflowing patient registry, while many of them are struggling just to stay afloat.

The Plight of the Cardiac Surgeon

Consider the CABG, for the last forty years the bread-and-butter operation for the average heart surgeon. During the decade 1993–2003, the number of CABGs in the United States declined about 11 percent, from about 340,000 to just over 300,000, even though the prime-age patient population grew by more than a fourth. Interventional cardiology, in the meanwhile, has been struggling with exploding workloads. Stents and angioplasties, the main catheter-based CABG substitutes, had more than doubled, to more than a million, by 2006. By 2000 or so, one- and two-coronary bypass operations were already becoming a rarity.

Rubbing it in, insurance reimbursement rates for CABGs have been steadily falling as well. Medicare reimbursement for the standard leg-vein triple-bypass operation is down 20 percent since 1998, or by about a third if inflation is taken into account. Private insurers pay better rates than Medicare, but the gap is narrowing fast as health plans consolidate and demand hospitalwide price concessions. Fees for interventional cardiologists have been dropping even faster than for heart surgeons, but soaring volumes more than make up the difference. Certainly, the TCT conference gave no hints of an embattled profession.

Postings on CTSNet, a Web site for cardiothoracic surgeons, are almost elegaic. Here's one from a surgeon in private practice in Missouri:

No jobs in Cardiac Surgery[?] Is this just a fallacy or is there any truth to it? Well, just look around and talk to your colleagues. . . . People are looking for jobs which are just not there at all, regardless of your training, years of research, graduating institution. . . . Obviously either the training was not adequate or the requirements of the market have changed. After an average of 10 years of cardiothoracic training, surgeons are opting to go for a second specialty training in anesthesia, vascular surgery and plastic surgery. The starting salary for [cardiac] surgeons is somewhere between $120,000 and $240,000, whereas an anesthesia graduate with a pain fellowship starts in the $400,000 range. [In some cases,] you are better off working at one of the larger institutions as a superfellow/adjunct-surgeon/instructor or even work as a physician assistant!. . . . A recently advertised job in South Florida offered the handsome compensation of $80,000/year for fully trained cardiac surgeons.

Signs that the wolf is really at the door came in the spring of 2006, when seventeen newly minted cardiothoracic surgeons failed to find jobs—the first time that has ever happened. The accreditation authorities responded by cutting back on accredited programs and residency slots. Worse, there is evidence that the best candidates may be drifting toward other specialties. Cardiothoracic residency slots have always drawn a surplus of candidates. But in the 2006 national residency match, there were only 102 applications for 126 approved slots. Eleven of the applicants then dropped out before the match, so 35 slots were not filled. That is unheard of—like Harvard going begging for undergraduate applications. The effect on academic program staffing will be profound. In the academic year 2004–2005, the first-year residency class was 141. In 2007–2008, when the group from the 2006 match begin their residencies, there will be only 91, a drop of 35 percent.

The relentless march of the cardiologists has not been without setbacks of its own. The first coronary "angioplasty" (or "vessel remolding") in a human took place in 1977. A catheter tube and balloon is threaded to the point of the occlusion, and the balloon is inflated to push the arterial walls open. It takes only an hour or so, usually with only local anesthesia. Patients go home the next day and are back to work a few days later—no chest scars, no months of recovery, no worry about bypass-machine neural effects. Angioplasty spread like wildfire. But as the case registry grew, the data showed a disturbing tendency toward reocclusion. So, yes, angioplasty is a patient-friendly way to reopen a coronary artery, but the odds are high that within a few years you'll need a do-over. With the CABG, by contrast, although the initial insult is much worse, the repair is closer to permanent. For most patients, the life-extension effects of the two procedures are roughly the same. Over time, cases with standard one- and two-vessel disease have migrated steadily to the cath lab—two or three redos over a decade or so isn't a bad tradeoff against a CABG. Three-vessel disease has mostly stayed in the CABG camp—three angioplasties imply a lot of redos—and there are subsets of patients, like diabetics and people with occlusions around the left ventricle, who clearly do better with the CABG. Cost differences are actually fairly modest—the initial angioplasty is much cheaper than a CABG, but the necessity for further interventions pushes total costs toward convergence.

The wire-mesh stent, unveiled in 1994, looked like a solution to the reocclusion problem. It is delivered folded around an angioplasty balloon and expanded within the occlusion to create a permanent scaffolding. But the stent's advantage over traditional angioplasties proved to be disappointingly modest. Yes, the scaffolding prevented the arterial walls from recollapsing, but the presence of the stent induces scar tissue proliferation, which is itself an important source of occlusions.

The drug-eluting stent—a stent coated with medication to prevent scar tissue formation—was the next breakthough, because it sharply reduced the rate of reocclusion. The DES, as it's called, burst on the scene in 2003, and by 2006 accounted for more than 80 percent of all U.S. stent placements. In just the three years since the FDA's approval of the first DES, a Johnson & Johnson product, the market exploded to annual sales of $6 billion, amid a colossal market slugfest between the two dominant players, J&J and Boston Scientific. With sales figures that rival those of blockbuster consumer drugs, DES is now the richest medical device market in history. I went to a conference in the spring where speakers confidently forecasted the near-term demise of the three-vessel CABG.

A few months before the 2006 TCT conference, how-ever, new data associated the DES with small, but statis-tically significant, increases in longer-term mortality. Excessive blood clotting in later years, it appears, may fully offset the benefits from low early reocclusion rates. One prominent cardiologist labeled the widespread use of DES "an epidemic of madness." By the spring of 2007, DES usage in the United States dropped from nearly 90 percent of all stents, by far the highest in the world, to about 70 percent, or about the same as in Japan. European stent usage, which was already low at 54 percent, dropped slightly to 51 per-cent, although there was wide variation from country to country. In December 2006, a divided FDA advisory com-mittee concluded that a DES was superior to a bare-metal stent for the relatively straightforward conditions approved by the FDA. For the more complex off-label uses—patients with long lesions, multivessel stenting, bifurcation (branch-ing) lesions, patients suffering from acute myocardial infarctions (heart attacks), and diabetics—that comprise the majority of DES placements, they agreed only that little was known of the efficacy and risks of DES compared to bare-metal stents or surgery. The panel also strongly recommended an extended anticlotting drug regimen for off-label patients and discouraged DES in patients who might have difficulty maintaining such a regimen.

The lavishness with which scientific brainpower and financial capital is being showered on the stent, however, as well as the large number of commercial teams working on the challenge, virtually ensure that stents will continue to expand their franchise. The cardiac surgeon who assumes his triple-bypass franchise is safe is reading the wrong tea leaves.

In the Cath Lab

After I had spent several months with the cardiac surgeons, I arranged with Marty Leon and Mat Williams to learn more about cath labs. At the time, Williams was assisting one of the senior cardiologists, Michael Collins, with diagnostic catheterizations. The "cath lab" looks like a mini-OR, but without the sterility trappings—for most procedures, everyone is in the usual OR scrubs, but there is no sterile field, no gowning, none of the obsessive elbow-deep prescrubbing. Inserting the typical cath looks much like giving blood at a Red Cross station. But while blood collection needles travel only a few inches into a vein, diagnostic catheters are threaded all the way into the heart, or liver, or other organ.

Every cath lab has an enormous assortment of guide wires and catheters arrayed along its walls. A routine angiogram usually requires the insertion of just a single catheter and guide wire, but in more complex procedures the guide wire may be left in place to facilitate access for a variety of other catheters and tools. Size, stiffness, outer coatings, may all vary depending on the instrument or the patient. There is considerable skill involved in advancing a catheter—how hard can I push in *this* patient to get around a difficult corner? Soft wires help in traversing sinuous regions, but stiffer wires may be needed to push through an occlusion. The shape of the catheter tips, the nature of the coatings, weight and stiffness, are the subject of intensive research. One firm advertises its products' superior "pushability."

The first diagnostic cath I saw was a straightforward

angiogram. The patient was being considered for a lung transplant, and Collins was just confirming that he had no coronary disease. The catheter was inserted into the left femoral (leg) artery in the groin area. From there it is a fairly straight shot through the right iliac artery, the abdominal aorta, the thoracic aorta—all just locational labels on the same giant pipeline—up to the aortic arch, then through the arch down to the aortic root and the junctures of the right and left coronary arteries. Soft tissues don't register on the imaging screen, so as Collins advanced the catheter, it appeared to float in a strange curving pattern through an empty rib cage, moving and bending of its own volition. While the image helped Collins fix his location, as an experienced interventionalist he could have done it by feel. At the aortic root, Collins rotated the catheter tip until he felt the entrance to the left coronary, inserted the catheter, squirted a dye, and froze the image as the dye flooded through the left-heart arterial network. He withdrew the catheter out of the left coronary, rotated it again, found the right coronary, and repeated the process. The coronaries looked fine.

The second procedure used a Swanz-Ganz catheter, a device that's been around since 1950. I'd seen the Swanz-Ganz before, since anesthesiologists use it to monitor cardiac flow dynamics in almost all open-heart surgeries. Collins's patient was an older woman with multiple comorbidities and progressive heart failure. The Swanz-Ganz has two blood-pressure sensors, one at the end and another further back, as well as a dilating balloon. It is usually inserted through the jugular, then follows the venous blood flow through the heart toward the lungs—

from the jugular to the vena cava, and through the right atrium and right ventricle into the pulmonary artery. In its final position, the intermediate sensor is in the right atrium, and the end-point sensor is in the pulmonary artery. In this case, Collins was primarily interested in the end-point measure. He inflated the balloon at the end-point sensor, briefly blocking blood flow through the pulmonary artery into the lungs, so the only pressure registering at the sensor was the backwash from the *lungs'* blood pressures. That was how the cardiologists in Iowa and St. Louis first identified Erika Maynard's pulmonary hypertension.*

The reading, as Collins had feared, showed pulmonary hypertension. He kept the catheter in place while he had the patient breathe pure oxygen, then, after waiting a bit, introduced a nitrous oxide (laughing gas) mixture and took another reading. If the lungs were at all reactive, the

---

*Notice that in measuring pulmonary hypertension, the backpressure into the blocked pulmonary artery is being used as a *proxy* for the pressure coming out of the lungs into the left atrium, which necessarily introduces some degree of error. To add to the uncertainty, the hypertensive index that transplant specialists use, the PVR (pulmonary vascular resistance), is a function of three variables, the (unblocked) pulmonary artery pressure, the so-called wedge pressure from the Swanz-Ganz described above, and cardiac output, which is based on yet another estimate. In the Maynard case, the surgeons later expressed considerable skepticism about Erika's near-miraculous PVR drop from close to 12 to only 1.7. Linda Addonizio, however, argues for its accuracy, based on the exceptional reactivity of pediatric cases, and the special skills in her section. The entire discussion is a good example of the fundamental imprecision of physiological indices, and the importance of experience and intuition in interpreting ostensibly precise data.

catheter would have registered a noticeable drop in pulmonary pressures. There was almost none at all. Collins looked sad. This was a very nice woman, he said, and he was going to have to tell her that she was going to die and that there was not much they could do for her. Her age, her physical condition, and the hypertension in the lungs pretty much ruled her out as a transplant candidate.

Later, I caught up with Leon to watch a stent placement. The patient had three blockages, but none in the major left-ventricle arteries, so he had opted for stents rather than a CABG. Leon started by threading two catheters into the right coronary. One was for angiogram dye, while the second placed the guide wire that would be used to transport the stents. He worked from two large imaging screens. When he squirted a bolus of dye, the right screen froze a shot of the bramble-bush layout of the patient's right coronaries, pinpointing the occlusions. The left screen was to track the stent catheter. As Leon worked the guide wire toward the first occlusion, it struck me what a remarkable feat of visual-tactile intelligence I was watching. Although everyone's coronary arteries follow roughly the same layout, the detailed branchings are unique. As he pushed the stent catheter, Leon could glance at the angiogram shot on the one screen and relate it to the wiggle pattern of the disembodied guide wire on the other, picking out turns mostly by the feel of the wire. Every couple of minutes, he'd pause for a pop of dye on the left-screen image to confirm that the wire was where he thought it was.

The first occlusion was a long one, located in a twisty byway, with a nearly right-angle turn in the center of the diseased section. For almost forty-five minutes, Leon pushed up, and then withdrew, several different stenting solutions. Drug-eluting stents are stiff, and he couldn't negotiate the turn with one of the proper length. He finally succeeded in placing two separate stents in the two legs of the right angle, eliciting quiet cheers from the whole team. The last two stent placements took only about five minutes, and the catheters were withdrawn, the wound bandaged, and the patient ready for transport within another quarter hour or so. Although the patient was sedated and drowsy, he was awake and communicative throughout the procedure.

The Cribier-Edwards Valve

Stan Rabinovich, voluble, rosy-cheeked, and grandfatherly, struck me as a happy man when I met him at his one-person office in Englewood, New Jersey. Rabinovich, along with Marty Leon and several other partners, was a founder of a company called PVT, in 1999. A couple of years before my visit, PVT had been purchased by the California-based Edwards Lifesciences, an important manufacturer of cardiology supplies, netting $6 million for each of the founding partners, along with the prospect of additional payments down the road. An extra fillip for Rabinovich is that Edwards has retained him as a one-man evangelist for the product he helped create, and which he loves to talk about—a catheter-delivered aortic valve replacement.

Rabinovich is an electrical engineer. Along with a friend, Stan Rowe, from Johnson & Johnson, he made major contributions to stent manufacturing. Rabinovich was sent to Paris in 1995 as head of J&J's European business development, where he met Alain Cribier, a well-known French cardiologist, who had pioneered the technique of "valvuloplasty"—the use of an angioplasty balloon to loosen and expand a calcifying aortic valve. Valvuloplasty was a disappointment, since so many valves quickly recalcified. Cribier had moved on to a valve replacement delivered "percutaneously" (doctor-Latin for "through the skin"—i.e., by means of a catheter). Rabinovich brokered a development agreement between Cribier and J&J.

Rabinovich and Rowe had both left J&J by 1999, when Rabinovich got a call from Cribier. Cribier told him that J&J "wasn't doing anything with his valve," and asked for his advice. Rabinovich and Rowe had met Leon when he was an outside medical director for J&J's interventional business, and took a train to Washington, where Leon practiced, to ask whether he thought Cribier's invention was a good idea. Leon thought it was a *very* good idea, and the three quickly formed a partnership with Cribier, who reacquired his rights from J&J. They put together a business plan and raised $500,000 from early-round "angel" investors, mostly through Leon's contacts in the medical community. Rabinovich and Rowe left their jobs and rented the one-room office where I met Stan. Impressively, they never hired other staff—no receptionist, no bookkeeper, no research assistants. The name PVT stood for Percutaneous Valve Technology.

They discovered they had a patent problem. A Danish doctor had patented a solution much like Cribier's in

1985, and his rights had been purchased by an American heart surgery company, Heartport, which had built a strong patent position. "We spent a long time analyzing the Heartport patents," Rabinovich said, "and finally decided there was no way around them." Heartport marketed tools and devices for performing heart surgery through small incisions. But they thought like surgeons, Rabinovich said, and gave up on the valve patent because they couldn't figure out how to remove the old valve. Cribier, by contrast, with his experience in valvuloplasty, left the old valve intact; he just expanded it with a balloon and put the new valve inside it. The pressure of the old valve ring would keep the new one in place while normal scar tissue created a permanent bond. Over a few hectic months, they struck a reasonable deal for the Heartport patent, located a high-tech contract manufacturer in Israel with good capabilities in materials sciences, and began developing valve prototypes. The technical challenges were formidable—the stent containing the valve in the current model is reputedly the strongest stent ever made.

PVT's world changed in 2002 when Cribier executed the first successful catheter-delivered aortic valve replacement in a human, working under a French "compassionate care" exception on a terminally ill patient who could never have survived standard surgery. Medical press front pages all around the world featured a picture of Cribier with his patient, who was smiling broadly and sitting up in bed, chest intact, drinking champagne within hours of receiving his new valve. Soon after, PVT executed a venture capital financing for $5 million, followed by a $14 million round that included industry heavy-hitters like

Medtronic. Buyout offers started in earnest in 2003, and a deal was done when Edwards showed up with a can't-refuse offer late in the year. Rowe is now running Edwards's valve business, while Rabinovich holds forth contentedly in Englewood. Not surprisingly, there are now dozens of companies working on a variety of aortic valve solutions, and nearly as much activity in mitrals, including some advanced work at Columbia.

An invasive heart device is subject to the same kind of rigorous approval processes as a new drug. At the time of the TCT conference, early-stage Cribier-Edwards trials throughout Europe and the United States had performed 282 procedures. Trial data were available only on the 55 cases conducted at Columbia-Presbyterian. Valves were successfully placed in 48, or 87 percent, of the patients, and the thirty-day mortality rate was 7.3 percent. That was more than double the most recent statewide mortality rate in surgical aortic valve replacement, but still a superb outcome, since the trial was limited to patients who were too sick or frail to tolerate standard surgery. Leon successfully placed a Cribier-Edwards valve in a hundred-year-old, as well as in several patients in their nineties.

I saw a Cribier-Edwards placement in April. Enthusiasm for the valve was building, so the operating area was unusually crowded—there was at least one team of observers from Europe, several senior figures from the hospital, people from Edwards, and probably others. The patient was a male, in his seventies, showing a reops' steel chest sutures on the imaging screen, who had been turned down for a surgical valve replacement. Leon and Moses were the interventionalists, with Mat Williams in attendance as well. The procedure took place in a cath lab, but one that was outfitted with most of the trappings of an OR—there was sterile field, the team was in sterile gowning, and the attending anesthesiologist, Sanford Littwin, was from the cardiac surgery anesthesiology team. I stayed in the windowed control room, which offered a good viewing perspective, with a complete bank of imaging screens, a microphone feed from the table, and a nurse–cardiology technician who was recording every step of the operation. It also happened to be one of the few operations that were unsuccessful, although it is a dramatic illustration of the procedural challenges.

To install the valve, the interventionalist first threads a balloon catheter from the femoral artery up through the aortal arch and into the valve. The balloon is pushed into the aortic valve and dilated—a valvuloplasty—to clear away calcification and expand the valve opening. In the case I saw, they did it twice. The balloon catheter is then withdrawn and replaced by the valve catheter. A challenging feature of the Cribier-Edwards procedure is that it requires an unusually large catheter payload. The patient I saw had a fairly large 26 mm valve opening. The Cribier-Edwards 26 mm valve-stent can be "crimped" down to about a third of that diameter, or just small enough to get through most adult male femorals. Once the new valve reaches the aorta, traverses the arch, and is positioned just above the old aortic valve, the patient's heart rate is electrically accelerated to about 200 beats per minute, inducing a fibrillation. Instead of beating, the heart just buzzes in place, so there is a stable catheter target. The new valve is quickly centered within the old one and expanded with a balloon to lock it into position. Then the balloon and catheter are withdrawn, and the pacing is decelerated back to a normal rate. The fibrillation lasts for only a half minute or so, which is reasonably safe.

In the case I saw, everything went as planned until the insertion of the valve catheter. This was a patient with extensive calcification in both femoral arteries, although one of them seemed clear enough for access. The valve catheter traversed the femoral smoothly, but got stuck on an outcropping of calcium in the iliac artery, around the mid-trunk area. Jeff Moses was inserting the catheter, and for several minutes he twisted or turned, angled and pushed it, but he couldn't clear the calcium. Then he withdrew the valve and dilated the calcified spot with a 10 mm balloon. (It's larger than cardiac catheter balloons and is normally used in non-cardiac vascular procedures.) When he reinserted the valve cath, it hung up for a few seconds at the calcified spot but, with a little pushing, suddenly released and sailed through, amid some back-slapping in the control room.

Then someone from the table said, "Arrest!" A glance at the EKG showed the heart beating, but blood pressure at zero. An injection of angiographic dye told the story—there was an evil plume of blood on the image screen, pouring out from the ruptured iliac like smoke from a burning building, right from the location of the calcification hang-up. One of the hospital's senior doctors, who had come down to the control room to greet the Europeans, put both hands on the table in front of him, closed his eyes and bowed his head.

Everyone in the room, I believe, thought they were witnessing a mortality. There had been several iliac ruptures in the European trials, and every one of the patients had died. This patient not only survived, but did so without apparent ill effects—a tribute to the skills of the people around the table. Somehow, Leon and Moses got another big balloon to the point of the rupture and blocked the bleeding. Littwin revved up the patient's blood pressure but managed not to dislodge the balloon. Williams did a fast cutdown to the site of the rupture, clamped it, and executed a rapid repair. Within the twenty minutes or so it took to ready a cardiac OR, the patient was already stabilized. Williams later told me that he worried that ischemia damage might require a leg amputation, but the patient was up and walking by the second day.

To my surprise, and to Marty Leon's infinite credit, I saw that same image again some months later at the TCT conference—the same dreadful shot of dark, dyed blood blowing out of a raggedly torn iliac—when he showed it to a room packed with about five hundred cardiologists. He had just completed a glowing account of the Cribier-Edwards trials—the high success rate, the stability of the valves, their excellent performance and tight sealing. Then he said, "Most people just like to show you what works. But I like to show everything that can go wrong." And he flashed up screen images of all of his failed cases, occasionally even lingering over them. "This is an extremely promising procedure," he concluded, "but it's not yet ready for general practice." There were a lot more trials to go, more work to be done on access methods, more development work on smaller, more "pushable" valve transporters. But there was no doubt that the craft of valve replacement was heading for radical change.

Meanwhile, Back at the OR

Not all the new developments are in the cath lab. In the spring, I arranged with Mike Argenziano to see a "robotic" surgery. The cardiologists had referred a patient with two diseased arteries—one they could stent, but the other, involving a large area of disease in a major left-side artery, required a bypass. Since the patient was hoping to avoid a sternotomy, it was agreed that the surgeons would do a minimally invasive off-pump bypass on the critical artery, while the cardiologists would stent the second artery a week or so later. Smith would execute the bypass, and Argenziano would harvest a mammary artery, using the da Vinci "robotic" surgical tool.

The da Vinci is a massive machine with two major components. The operating unit, which comes on heavy wheels and is more than six feet high, is positioned at the foot of the operating table. It has up to four large, praying mantis–type stainless-steel arms with a video display at the center. The control unit is about the size of a large armchair and is positioned off to the side of the OR. The surgeon sitting at the console can control any of the arms through two control knobs, while watching what he's doing on the console's 3-D, high-definition color screen. The table team can also follow the surgery through table video display.

The two critical features of the da Vinci are the 3-D picture—depth-perception mistakes in surgery can be disastrous—and the "endo-wrist" knob system. The knobs transmit the surgeon's actual wrist and finger motions to the remote tools, in user-selected transmission ratios. Argenziano sets his at 3:1—a 3 mm turn of his wrist turns the tool 1 mm, while squeezing index finger and thumb will open and close the blades of a scissors one-third that much. (Smith, characteristically, sets his at 1:1.)

I came into the OR when Argenziano was setting up the da Vinci. He was being helped by a woman—in her late thirties, I guessed—wearing green OR scrubs rather than Columbia-Presbyterian's light blue. Her name was Felicia Brodzky, and she was the local da Vinci account manager. We met for coffee a few days later, and she explained that she spent her workday traveling from OR to OR throughout Manhattan, helping surgeons with the da Vinci. Her boss would prefer that she wear a business suit, but she said she saved a lot of time by wearing scrubs to work, partly to avoid all the changing, but also because security staff automatically wave through people in scrubs—a trick I had figured out by then too. She wasn't a medical professional, but her undergraduate work was in science, and she was clearly very knowledgeable about surgery. In the two da Vinci procedures I saw, she was very useful, jumping in when a resident got confused during a tool change, for instance. Her company is doing well, and I imagine she is well paid.

Argenziano used three of the arms for the arterial harvest —one for a camera, and two for tools. The knob settings are adjustable, so either one can control any of the tools. The resident made three quarter-inch incisions around the patient's chest and inserted a tool arm through each one. Then the patient's chest was inflated with gas to increase the working space, and the operation proceeded as normal. Argenziano arguably had better visualization of his target vessel than he would in an open-chest operation, he could zoom his vision field in and out as he needed to, and he had extremely fine, tremor-free control over his instruments. The functionings of the da Vinci that were not directly related to the surgery—like getting the arms positioned at setup—struck me as a bit clunky, and the size and expense of the machine makes it a difficult purchase, but the surgery itself proceeded beautifully. There was a good selection of tools, and Argenziano could cut, clamp, grasp, and stitch virtually any way he pleased. When he finished, the mammary had been cleanly harvested and clamped, and was lying on the pericardium for Smith's bypass.*

The minimally invasive bypass was routine. Argenziano cut a four-inch incision between two ribs, which he spread with a miniretractor, but without breaking them, and

---

*The initial market penetration of the da Vinci, it appears, has been in areas where laparascopic procedures are well established. (They are small-incision, camera-assisted surgeries, usually in the belly.) Surgeons used to laparoscopic techniques usually find that the 3-D, highly intuitive character of the da Vinci is a big improvement over laparoscopy, and requires minimum adaptation on their part. It is also becoming the technology of choice for prostate surgery, since the fine-grained control substantially enhances preservation of sexual and urinary functions. The gas pressure within the abdomen also reduces bleeding. Unlike most prostatectomies, a urologist told me, da Vinci prostatectomies rarely require blood transfusions. Amid all this good news, the company, unfortunately, is increasing its prices to well over a million dollars for a basic system. If the history of computer hardware is any guide, the victor in robotic surgery will be the company that produces a highly functional, compact, low-priced system that becomes standard in every OR in the world, not the one selling a "mainframe" solution. Finally, the da Vinci is not in any sense robotic—it is a servo-mechanism—but the "robotic" tag has stuck, and is a great attention-getter.

Smith used a long set of tools to execute an off-pump bypass. The bypass itself probably took a little longer than a single open-chest bypass would have done, but the overall savings, in chest opening and closing, trauma recovery, and bypass machine side effects, must have been immense. This was also the first time I'd seen Argenziano's "A-rod" in action. It is a rodlike tool he invented to stabilize a coronary artery during a minimally invasive off-pump operation, and the name both reflects his authorship and proclaims his favorite Yankee player. A major surgical supplier carries the A-rod in its catalog.

In December 2006, a new set of trials on the Cribier-Edwards valve got under way that illustrates one path of convergence between heart surgery and interventional cardiology. The FDA authorized a preliminary set of twenty "transapical" Cribier-Edwards placements. The principal investigators, effectively the trial managers, are Marty Leon and Craig Smith, and the procedures will be carried out at Columbia-Presbyterian, the Cleveland Clinic, and Medical City Dallas Hospital. In a transapical placement, the surgeon makes a mini-incision in the lower chest, places a purse-string suture* in the apex, or bottom point, of the heart, and inserts a catheter. The interventionalist

---

*The "purse-string suture," which is the standard method of inserting a tube into an organ, is just one of dozens of high-efficiency surgical techniques that have evolved from long practice. The surgeon places a suture in a circle around the area of incision, with the two ends coming together, as in the top of a sack. The incision is made *after* the suture is in place. In almost a single motion, a skilled surgeon can make the incision, insert the tube, and pull the purse-string shut, so there is almost no loss of blood. When it's time to extubate, he pulls out the tube, tightens the purse-string, and ties it shut.

then threads the catheter through the left ventricle to the aortic valve, performs the balloon valvuloplasty, and places the new valve.

The transapical procedure potentially offers multiple advantages. The access route is much shorter, with no concerns over access-route diameters. Unlike the procedure I saw, in which the valve was inserted through an artery to the aorta, or against the direction of the blood flow, the transapical approach follows the blood flow through the ventricle and enters the valve from the bottom, so there should be fewer problems with flow turbulence and less chance of getting stuck on a partially open valve. The first two placements at Columbia-Presbyterian went smoothly. They took place in the new hybrid OR. Mat Williams was the interventionalist and Allan Stewart the surgeon, with Smith, Moses, and Leon all in attendance.

Managing Convergence

In a rational world, professional guilds would organize around diseases and treatments, not around methods of access. But when the favored method of access is the full sternotomy—which is a bit like getting hit by a cruise missile—it will tend to dominate the conversation. But as surgery becomes less traumatic, and interventional cardiology more aggressive, boundaries based on access modes should diminish. Mat Williams's joint appointment harbingers a new breed of cardiac specialists who can offer patients a menu of choices without regard to guild distinctions. A conference on valve repair would draw valve specialists who offer the full range of techniques from tool-boxes we now label "surgical" or "interventionalist."

When I spoke to Williams about convergence issues, he made the important point that different approaches come with different success standards. "If you do a transcatheter mitral repair," he said, "you might be satisfied with a two-plus regurge [an index of valve leakage]. At that level, a lot of people are asymptomatic. But you would never dream of ending an open-chest procedure with a valve like that. If a patient goes through a chest opening and a bypass, he has a right to a regurgitation of zero." That suggests new possibilities in adapting solutions to patient needs. For many, an adequate, but imperfect, result from a low-stress procedure will be a best-case outcome. When it's not, you can move on to more invasive approaches. "The important thing," Williams said, "is not to destroy the bridge to surgery. If your simple procedure would make it impossible to repair the valve surgically later on, then you shouldn't do it."

The likely migration path toward the cardiac-interventionalist specialty will probably be from the surgical ranks. For one thing, that's where the manpower surpluses are, but the surgical craft disciplines also take longer to learn. "The general surgery residency lets you develop skills working on low-pressure operations like hernias," Williams said, "but there is no easy cardiac surgery." When the Cribier-Edwards valve is inserted through the femoral, he went on, you need a surgeon to close the wound, since it's bigger than the one an ordinary cath needle makes. "It's a simple procedure," he said, "and a cardiologist could learn how to do it, but it wouldn't make much sense. If something went wrong, he'd suddenly be facing a major artery repair and would be in very deep trouble."

However smoothly the reconfiguring of the profession proceeds over the long term, the near- and medium-term challenges will be very daunting. Leading-edge heart centers like Columbia-Presbyterian have been able to maintain their case volumes by radically diversifying their practices and developing a steady stream of new techniques and procedures—aortic and mitral valve repair, valve-sparing aortic root replacement, a variety of new approaches to aneurysms and to fibrillation, new heart-assist devices, breakthroughs in congenital surgery, and much more. But as the kit bag of surgical interventions expands, only the largest centers can maintain adequate volumes in a good cross-section of interventions. Even now, many surgeons in community practice rarely see a valve case. Consider some of the implications:

+ The large centers will continue to take case share, while medium and small centers will lose volumes. Skills and safety will deterioriate. Should they be closed down?
+ As programs fall away, will large swathes of the country be left without cardiac surgeons to intervene in heart attacks? And who will provide the surgical backup for the interventional cardiologists?
+ If residencies are curtailed—either by policy or by lack of interest—how will the teaching hospitals make up the staff losses?

✦   And what will happen ten to fifteen years from
now, when the baby boomers hit their seventies
and start needing a lot more heart surgery?

These are very difficult issues, of the kind that the professional societies and accreditation bodies are not well equipped to deal with. The natural leadership of the profession, moreover, is centered in the big universities, and is remote from the problems of community surgeons. It is a profession, in short, that is facing interesting times.

Chapter 9

MONEY

Top academic surgeons are well paid. Columbia University's 2004 tax returns showed that Eric Rose earned $2.0 million; Mehmet Oz, $1.6 million; and Craig Smith, $1.5 million.* Top doctors can also earn substantial outside income as speakers, consultants, and board members. Rose is a director of several outside companies, while Oz has a strong income stream from his books. (Total U.S. sales of his *You: The Owner's Manual,* a *New York Times* number-one best-seller, was about 1.6 million through the end of 2006, while his new book, *You: On a Diet*, released in November 2006, jumped to the top of the best-seller lists

*Nonprofit tax returns are available to the public and must list the entity's top five earners. Previous years' returns show that Jan Quaegebeur's earnings were usually right behind Smith's. Jeffrey Moses, the director of the interventional cardiology division came to Columbia in 2004, however, and, at $2.2 million, pushed Quaegebeur off the list. The top-earning Columbia physician in recent years has been a dermatologist, David Silvers, who earned an impressive $3.6 million in 2004.

its first week, with 2,000,000 copies in print. Both books are coauthored with Dr. Michael F. Roizen.) Smith does not have outside income, which makes him something of a throwback. Earnings of the younger attendings apparently cluster around the mid–six figures, with a healthy tilt toward the upper end of that range.

The cardiothoracic division is a unit of the Columbia Medical School and the surgeons are university employees. They are paid modest faculty salaries plus "additional income," from their surgical fees, after covering the division's overhead costs. The surgical infrastructure—ORs, OR equipment, recovery rooms, nurses, physicians' assistants, and the like—is operated and financed by New York–Presbyterian Hospital from hospital charges. The precise line between divisional and hospital costs is a matter for multiple annual minibargains—since cardiac surgery is among the more profitable services, the hospital is often willing to pick up divisional costs to increase patient throughput. The splits of the "additional income" among the surgeons and other staff are handled within the division. Smith told me they had struggled to come up with performance-based formulas, but now he just makes the allocations himself. No one has complained: he is known to be fair, and doesn't take the biggest share.

I could not find a data source for private-practice heart surgeon income. Best estimates from several senior surgeons on a 2005 medical student Web forum converged in the $300,000-to-$800,000 range. Given the steady contraction in CABGs, however, and the increasing proportion of complex cases that require large-center infrastructures, there seems little doubt that surgeons in outlying areas and smaller hospitals are being squeezed. But at the same time, elite private-practice cardiac surgeons may be doing better than ever, far better than even the Roses and Smiths of the world, especially if they own and operate a specialty hospital—typically a forty-to-fifty-bed for-profit center optimized for state-of-the-art, but mostly routine, cardiac procedures. The special-service focus generates higher operating margins than at a general hospital or an academic center, and the doctor-owners collect both the hospital charges and the surgical fees. Specialty hospitals are controversial, since they allegedly "cream off" the most profitable patients from community hospitals and, some worry, create inherent conflicts of interest for the physician-owners; but no one denies that they generally provide good-quality care.

Are heart surgeons overpaid? A New York newspaper published the Columbia-Presbyterian 2002 salaries with the clear implication that they were too high, especially for a nonprofit institution. But by New York City standards, $1 to $2 million a year is not an especially impressive income. Youthful bond traders and investment bankers, law firm partners, commercial real estate brokers, generally make at least as much and frequently much more, sometimes ten, twenty, even a hundred times more. I am writing this chapter a few weeks after watching Yoshi Naka and Mo Garrido work intensely for nearly eight hours to place an LVAD so that an elderly man could have a couple more years of a reasonably normal life. Investment bankers and lawyers will tell you that they work hard too. But Naka and Garrido were on their feet, hunched over the table the entire period, with no breaks for food, water, or bathroom. They are also one of the relatively few teams in the world who can do such operations. Garrido was in his fourteenth year of postcollege training and was making less than a kid fresh out of law school doing case research at a New York firm. Naka may have been in the range of a midlevel law partner. These guys are not overpaid.

Becoming "Businesslike"

One sign of the times is the way business jargon is seeping into the medical vocabulary. I heard surgeons refer to their patients as "customers," and their procedures as "products" they were selling in "markets." And, indeed, while surgery and the teaching of surgery is an art form, decisions about running a surgical unit and deciding where to invest and whom to hire are much like those in any business. From the months I spent at Columbia-Presbyterian, I extracted four "business cases," as M.B.A.'s call them. They are: introducing a new "product," adding a new "business line," upgrading "customer care," and billing and collecting. Overall, I think they capture the blurry overlap between the craft ethos of the surgeons and the commercial aspects of their practice—perhaps what one would expect of a university faculty that happens to have large cash flows.

New Product. Allan Stewart is the youngest attending. He was just a year out of his residency when I first met him, but has already built Columbia-Presbyterian into a national center for specialized aortic surgery. He comes from a middle-class family but, as the second of five children, financed much of his higher education with loans and scholarships. After attending Saint Peter's College in Jersey City, he did his medical school training at the New Jersey College of Medicine, which operates a shambolic general hospital in one of the poorer areas of Newark. The hospital was "in ruins," he said, but the hyperactive emergency room was a great introduction to hands-on, crisis-oriented medical and surgical interventions. By all accounts, Stewart is a gifted surgeon, and he must have distinguished himself in Newark, for his next stop was a top-flight surgical residency at the University of Pennsylvania, and then to Columbia, where he became something of a Smith protégé.

At the end of his cardiothoracic residency, Stewart signed on for an additional six months in LVADs, partly to decompress and partly to have more free time to job-hunt. LVADs are a low-volume procedure, so he also did a lot of operations as an attending surgeon. A break came when he covered for Smith during the summer vacation period and got a series of referrals for aortic valves and aortic aneurysms (a kind of hernia in the wall of the aorta). Cardiologists who had been pleased with his work kept sending him cases, and by fall he was building a modest aortic practice of his own. "I didn't have an assigned OR," he said, "so I had to pick up a room however I could—cancellations, Saturdays, Sundays, that kind of thing. And I wasn't getting paid anything besides my residency salary"—although, with two young kids, he sometimes had difficulty explaining those financial arrangements to his wife.

By fall, however, Stewart was getting attractive job

offers. "Craig would always trash them," he said. "Why would you want to live in New Mexico? But by November, my wife is saying, 'Look, we're going to have to relocate in two months, and we have no idea where we're going to go! Your kids won't have any health insurance!' Then Craig came by one day and said, 'You've been building this aortic practice—would you like to stay?' And I said yes. We never talked about money." The division did not have a strong aortic practice outside of valves, so Stewart and Smith agreed that's where he would focus his attention.

Stewart's reputation and referral base both grew rapidly. He is one of only about a half dozen or so U.S. surgeons who do "valve-sparing root replacements." The aortic root is the bottom of the aorta, where it connects to the heart and encloses the aortic valve. Since root aneurysms usually pull apart the valve, the standard procedure is to replace the entire root with a prosthesis containing a new mechanical valve and a synthetic reinforcing wall for the aneurysm. Stewart still repairs the aneurysm in the usual way, but first usually repairs the natural valve, which almost always works out better for the patient than a manufactured valve. (I didn't see an actual operation, but did see a slide presentation. It's clearly very tricky.) I asked him how he learned the procedure. He said, "I did a lot of reading, and saw a couple videos by the man who invented it, and I practiced a lot on hearts we'd removed from transplant patients. And by now I've developed wrinkles of my own." Inevitably, much richer offers started coming in from other heart centers. Smith did another stroll-by and asked if he'd stay if they doubled his salary. "I said yes," Stewart smiled.

"It's true that you can make more in private practice," he went on, "but I make enough money. And I love academic medicine. I like doing the undoable operations, the high-risk surgery, the case that's been turned down by two other surgeons, and the patient comes in and says, I want to live, can you help me? It makes me happy. I don't want to do one routine triple-bypass after another so guys can get back to their golf games. And I love the teaching. You're also better supported in academic medicine, so I can have something like a normal family life."

The very uncommercial, almost casual, approach to what became a very profitable undertaking seems typical of the way the division does its business. No one drew up an "aortic business plan," laid out the finances, or developed a billing strategy. It was some time, in fact, before Stewart learned that he wasn't billing correctly for his valve-sparing root procedure. "At first, I billed it as a standard root replacement," he said. "I didn't realize that it qualified both as a valve repair and a new root." That's how academics think.

New Business Line. I took a predawn charter flight with Craig Smith one spring morning to sit in on an 8 A.M. M&M and case review meeting with the cardiac team at the Arnot Ogden Medical Center in Elmira, New York. There were about a dozen people at the meeting, including the local cardiac surgeons, several cardiologists, and other cardiac staff. Substantively, the meetings were much like the ones at Columbia, although doubtless because of Smith's presence as an external eminence, they were somewhat more formal and the cases more thickly documented, with less of the fast-fire verbal shorthand that the Columbia surgeons used. When the M&Ms were finished, the Elmira doctors reviewed the treatment plans for several borderline cases with Smith. (He was characteristically thorough, but agreed with them all and told me later that the current team was quite good.) After Smith arranged for one of the Elmira surgeons to come to Columbia for a refresher in vascular surgery, we headed to the airport and were back at the hospital before 10:30 A.M.

Arnot Ogden was one of eight cardiothoracic contractual "affiliates" as of the end of 2006. Three of them were in New York, two in New Jersey, two in Virginia, and one in South Carolina. The first such agreement was executed in 1997 and Arnot Ogden, the second, was signed two years later. At least a couple of the affiliations were prompted by regulatory concerns about a cardiac practice going offtrack. The contracts are coordinated on a consultancy basis by Paul Kurlansky, a semiretired cardiothoracic surgeon who trained at Columbia-Presbyterian. When I first met Kurlansky, he had just returned from Connecticut, where he had been evaluating the physical plant at a hospital that was opening a new cardiac surgery center. The hospital had sought a relationship with Columbia-Presbyterian to help them navigate the operational start-up and stabilization.

Kurlansky, whose primary job is research director at the Florida Heart Research Foundation, is usually most heavily involved in getting a new affiliation agreement off the ground. Along with Larry Beilis, the operations manager for the Department of Surgery, he works out a financial and marketing plan, reviews the facilities, and assists in capital planning, much like any business consultant. Since

Kurlansky is an experienced hand at clinical trials, he can also assist affiliates in becoming trial sites, often a good device for capturing the attention of local cardiologists.

One of the great benefits for an affiliate, besides the Columbia oversight, is that their key surgeons get Columbia faculty status, and Columbia-Presbyterian will recruit the chief, which greatly expands the recruitment pool. Affiliate faculty don't teach at Columbia, but they have video-feed access to Columbia faculty meetings, which helps them stay abreast of the field. They are also welcome in the Columbia-Presbyterian ORs to observe new techniques and tools.

To get a more concrete picture of the workings of an affiliate arrangement, I visited one at the University Hospital in Newark where Allan Stewart had trained. The cardiac chief, Barry Esrig, was a regular attendee at the Columbia faculty meetings, and also did occasional transplant duty and helped with resident training, but his workdays were spent in Newark. This is a hospital that for years has been notorious for poor quality, and they had reached out to Columbia in a last-ditch effort to save their program. Esrig is a native New Yorker, in his early sixties; he did his cardiothoracic residency at Montefiore Medical Center in the Bronx, then spent seventeen years in private practice in Los Angeles.

Esrig said that he enjoyed life as a private practitioner, and did well financially, but he also missed the academic environment—the greater number of challenging cases and the daily interactions with quality people. He got an appointment as a voluntary faculty member at UCLA, then spent three years on the full-time faculty at the University of Southern California. He was looking for an opportunity to return to New York when a mutual friend recommended him to Smith, who was just then trying to staff out an affiliate agreement.

University Hospital was Esrig's second affiliate assignment. The first one was a smaller Newark hospital with a cardiac program that he said was a "disaster," much as University was. In both cases, all the surgeons were outsiders, and no one was managing the program. "So there were no protocols in the OR," he said, "no postoperative protocols, and none in the ICU—and no separate cardiac ICU at all. Everyone had a different instrument table, the nurses were't trained in cardiac, the anesthesiologist was self-taught." In both cases, he said, "mortality was very high."

At his first affiliate, Esrig said, "I made a point of scrubbing with each of the surgeons, and I remember showing one senior man the newer methods for protecting the heart during an operation. He listened very patiently, and then he said, "Thank you very much, young man, that was very interesting, but would you please now step aside so I can do my case the way I prefer to."

What was Esrig's recipe for turning around a cardiac surgery program? "The first thing is to hire a good anesthesiologist," he said. At his first affiliate, his Columbia colleagues recommended one of their own, an experienced man named Doug Jackson, who later also transferred with him to University. "Doug not only brought good anesthesiology," Esrig said, "but he created the protocols we needed in the ORs and in the ICU, and he could train the nurses. Then I had to build a minimum infrastructure—a separate coronary ICU, with separate staff—and create protocols and clinical pathways that were enforced, plus computers, data collection, in-service training, case reviews." He went on: "Everyone knows about the relationship between high volumes and good outcomes, but it's not just because of the volumes themselves. High-volume places are forced to nail down all their supporting processes, and have reliable, well-trained people at every stage. Otherwise, you couldn't keep up. What I basically did was to replicate high-volume methods in a low-volume center." The last step was to quietly squeeze out the poor-performing doctors. "Everybody knows who they are, but patients often love them. The administrators backed me at both sites, however, and we didn't embarrass anyone. It was all done very quietly."

In his first affiliate, Esrig said, all the external measures turned around quickly, but the affiliation ended when Columbia-Presbyterian asked for full control over the unit's hiring and firing, which the hospital didn't want to concede. But they did hire an excellent full-time director, Esrig said, and the program continues in good shape.

The record at University was much the same. In three years, mortality rates dropped from a catastrophic 6.63 percent to only 0.83 percent, one of the lowest in the state and about half the state average. The last review from the accreditation authorities was almost a hymn of praise. One reviewer wrote that he "had rarely seen so substantial and dramatic an improvement" in a surgical program. (Giving all credit to the operational improvements Esrig made, however, the fact that Esrig was doing a disproportionate share of the surgery clearly accounted for much of the improvement. Methods are important, but they don't trump good surgeons.) Despite the improvement, the training program will shut down anyway. With the compression of the cardiac surgery job market, the accreditation authorities are ending most small programs, and because of its history, University was an obvious early choice.

The affiliation agreements generate welcome revenue at a time when fees of all kinds are being cut, and they clearly qualify as a successful entrepreneurial initiative. The organizational model the affiliation assumes—a hub-and-spoke model of outlying surgical operations linked to a center of excellence—also makes sense in a world of very rapid technological change. Still, I was struck by the very large element of happenstance in its origins and development. It was not a separate unit or "profit center" as it would have been in most business settings. Smith clearly spent a lot of time on it, but there was no full-time director, or any concerted effort to market the service, no overall "affiliation business plan" or revenue objectives. Instead, the work was divided up informally among all the attendings, and issues were thrashed out by the whole group, much like any other special project of a university faculty.

Customer Care. One area where business thinking has made a clear impact is in "customer care" practices. Patients generally get to heart surgeons only through a cardiologist's referral. By the time of a patient's first appointment at the cardiothoracic division, the surgeon and cardiologist will have discussed the case, gone over the records, possibly ordered additional tests, and usually agreed on a course of action. Sometimes patients want to think about the surgery after they meet the surgeon, but as often as not, their minds are already made up and a full case-intake process happens on the first day. It can, indeed, take most of a day—besides the surgical interview, there are numerous forms to fill out, possibly more tests, meetings with a hospital cardiologist, an anesthesiologist, a division social worker–educator, and possibly others.

I sat in on several patient meetings, with the surgeons, the anesthesiologists, and the educator. My first reaction was surprise that they were almost all on time or very close to it. Partly that was due to the top-drawer divisional administrative and clerical staff—they work hard, appear to take lunch at their desks most days, are invariably polite and friendly, and either answered patient questions on the spot or tracked down the answers. (They are also paid well, and the division's surgical fees fund bonuses for good performers.) The doctors, unlike those in my past experience, had clearly internalized the importance of a decent customer experience, and reflexively apologized if an appointment started late, even just five to ten minutes late.

The extra touches seemed mostly the work of Diane Amato, the cardiac division administrator (a title that does not begin to encompass her duties). She is a warm, empathetic woman who has been with the unit for eighteen years and has clearly worked hard to simplify the process for patients. She conducts a number of the educational interviews—one of the last pieces of the intake process. The purpose of the meeting is to answer any lingering questions on the operation and to walk the patient through exactly what would happen on the day of surgery. At the end, she gives the patient a large plastic carrying bag. Besides written instructions and assorted tschotkes, like antibacterial soap for the night-before shower, it contains a large placard and a track suit in Columbia blue and white. The placard is for the patient's car windshield: they can just leave their car at the hospital's main entrance and staff will look after it. The track suit is the cardiac surgery uniform: security staff will recognize wearers as cardiac patients, wave them past any waiting lines, and make sure they get to where they're supposed to be. "You and your family will have enough on your minds that morning," Amato tells them. "You shouldn't have to hunt for parking or wait in security lines."

Billing and Collection. The cardiothoracic division's billing and collection group is one of the very few that has not been subsumed by the hospital's central billing unit. "We know the patients," Amato said, "and collect a much higher percentage of charges than a central unit ever could." It's worth it to maintain their own unit, she says, although the hospital still assesses the division with its share of the central unit's cost.

I spent a couple of hours with Amato and her billing team. The division has contracts with a handful of major insurance plans, and also takes Medicare and Medicaid patients. (Some hospital divisions no longer accept Medicare. Congress generally expands Medicare services faster than its revenue base. To make ends meet, Medicare fees have been steadily cut, and are now almost always much lower than private insurance rates.) In all, the division collects from as many as 2,800 different payer groups, although a small percentage of those make up the bulk of all collections.

Hospital billing has long since entered a shadow world

of pseudorationality. "Usual and customary," or posted, fees are virtually meaningless. Medicare rates are established by federal authorities at only a small fraction of the posted rates. Medicaid is a joint federal-state program, with rates even lower than Medicare's. The private-plan contracts—the "in-plan" payers—pay against individually negotiated rate schedules that are usually higher than Medicare's, but still only a fraction of the posted rates. Finally, "out-of-plan" rates are negotiated case by case for patients whose insurers don't have hospital contracts. Out-of-plan rates are almost always higher than the in-plan rates, although still not at posted levels.

Out-of-plan patients make up a substantial portion of the caseload, and must accept personal payment responsibility at the *posted* rate. From what I could see, almost all patients agree to pay, although many of them would certainly have difficulty coming up with the $50,000-to-$100,000 or so cost of a major operation and recovery. After the surgery, the division expects the patient to cooperate in pursuing a claim with the out-of-plan carrier and in almost all cases the division negotiates a reasonable payment. But that money is paid to the patient, not to the hospital, so there still may be a difficult collection involved. If the patient promptly turns over the payment, plus a reasonable copayment, the bill is treated as paid. If the patient does not cooperate in pursuing the claim, or doesn't turn over the funds received, the division will use commercial bill collectors, who target their collections at the posted rate.

One case is something of a local classic. An out-of-plan patient had a major, and successful, congenital repair operation, received a very large payment from his carrier, and blew it on an extravagant family party. After a few attempts at collection, the division dropped the case. A few years later, the patient brought in a child with the same problem. Amato made sure all the surgeons understood the history before they took the new case, but they took it anyway. This time, in fact, when the former patient collected the nonplan payment, he not only turned it over to the hospital, but he and the family began a payment plan against the first fee as well. The willingness of the surgeons to take the case didn't surprise me, since I had seen collections questions come up at attendings meetings. The surgeons were usually worried that the division was dunning patients, while Amato was usually pleading with the surgeons not to tell their patients that they really didn't have to pay.

There is a strongly held opinion, particularly among conservative think tanks, that with multiple competitive private payers, the normal interactions between vendors and payers will gradually create a more efficient health care system. I saw no evidence to support that belief. What actually happens is that Smith and the billing staff sit down each year, lay out the various payment plans on a spreadsheet, and decide on the division strategy—which surgeons will join which plans, and which carriers will be carried on a nonplan basis, trading higher payments for greater collection risk. Once that strategy is set, it is managed entirely by the collections staff. The surgeons simply join the plans they're assigned to.

It is an interesting collision, I think, between two quite rational, but alien, thought systems. Classical market economists tend to define rationality as maximizing economic outcomes. The division's equally rational strategy is to *neutralize* the plethora of payment incentives so the surgeons can practice their craft according to their lights, with minimum economic penalty.

This is a contest that the surgeons will almost always win. Health care pricing doesn't work like a grain auction. The terms of insurance company health plans are set bureaucratically and changed only infrequently, with very little feedback on actual vendor behavior. And the plans are so complex, and the course of a difficult case so unpredictable, that it is often impossible to know in advance what a final price will be. For all those reasons, game theory would suggest that the surgeons' "neutralization" strategy is the sensible choice. It is not that classical economics has no relevance to big-ticket health care—the proliferation of specialty hospitals suggests otherwise. But it is not the dominant paradigm or, within the Columbia-Presbyterian cardiothoracic division, even a particularly important one. In other words, attempting to reenvision big-ticket medicine as a conventional problem in microeconomics may be what Alfred Whitehead called a "category error."

Advancing the Field

Columbia is also a research university, and as in all universities, the surgeons' advancement up the academic ladder depends heavily on the amount and quality of original work they do.

Henry Spotnitz, the vice chairman for research in the

Department of Surgery, is a cardiothoracic surgeon whose practice has recently been concentrated in pacemakers and defibrillators, two of his research specialties. He is perhaps best known, however, for some thirty years' work elucidating the anatomy and workings of the left ventricle —painstakingly building a picture of the changes in internal volumes, wall thicknesses, and other geometries over a heartbeat cycle, all crucial background for understanding the heart's internal flow dynamics.

At first glance, the research output expected of the surgical faculty seems astonishingly high—at least three major papers a year for an assistant professor, Spotnitz said, or about three times that in most academic departments. But surgeons are mostly doing "translational," rather than fundamental research. The business definition of research and development, or R&D, classifies work in basic science under the R, while specific product development is part of the D. On that definition, Spotnitz said, the surgeon's research was much more on the D side.

Most surgical papers, in fact, flow directly from ongoing work in the OR. Allan Stewart, for example, told me he was preparing a paper on the modifications he has made in valve-sparing root procedures, and a second one as principal surgical investigator on the Cribier-Edwards percutaneous valve that Marty Leon demonstrated at the TCT conference (Chapter 8). For his third, he is part of an LVAD team research effort for a paper slated to be published in *Nature*, one of the highest-prestige journals, on tissue reactions to continuous-flow LVAD pumps (Chapter 4). The *Nature* paper will be the first of two, with the second one focusing on chemical changes.

Spotnitz ran through some highlights of recent Columbia faculty research. Smith has done a lot of work in valves, minimally invasive procedures, and cardio protection through hypothermia (cooling) and the application of cardioplegia. Rose is a leading figure in LVAD research, while Oz has made a range of contributions in LVADs, minimally invasive procedures, arrhythmias, atrial fibrillations, and angiogenesis (encouraging the growth of new cardiac blood vessels). Argenziano's work has concentrated in robotics, minimally invasive procedures, and valves, and Stewart's in valves and the aorta. The pediatric side, especially Quaegebaer, has made many contributions to congenital surgery, as have Quaegebaer and Mosca in understanding arrhythmias, while Jonathan Chen has a recent *Nature* paper on LVADs. Mat Williams will be focusing on percutaneous and surgical valve replacements and repairs.

The bench laboratory research to support these programs is conducted in a rabbit warren of offices with the disorderly confusion of computers, test equipment, lab vials, and bottles of mysterious fluids that seem to mark all biotech labs. The division also has animal laboratories —much of Spotnitz's ventricular research was done on dogs—while most of the percutaneous experiments are conducted in the new animal ORs at Marty Leon's Cardiovascular Research Foundation about a half hour upstate from the university.

Most of the detailed bench work is executed by research assistants—generally surgical residents doing a research year, medical students, plus a smattering of undergraduate interns, supported by a mixture of NIH grants, a tax on surgical earnings, foundation support, and industry support. Medtronic makes a small contribution to Spotnitz's research in cardiac electrophysiology, but most industry support is tied to trials of new devices or tools.

In June 2006, I sat in on a meeting between Mehmet Oz and a mostly new crop of lab assistants. (This was the meeting where he gave each new assistant a copy of Strunk and White's *Elements of Style* and delivered a homily on the professional importance of learning how to write clearly.) The two senior researchers were Tim Martens and Mark Russo, both of them taking a break from Columbia surgical residencies. I had met Russo on an organ harvest trip (Chapter 4), and he has since rejoined his surgical residency program. Martens is using his break from surgery to complete a Columbia Ph.D. in bioengineering, which he somehow manages to coordinate with his lab work. Both plan to go on to cardiothoracic programs when they complete their general surgical residencies. The other assistants were a polyglot group from all over the world—Oz makes a practice of giving smart kids with no connections a shot at the fast track.

The active projects included several on the generation of new heart vessels with adult bone marrow stem cells, a follow-up study of "bow-tie" mitral repair (a minimally invasive procedure partly developed by Oz), several transplant follow-up studies, follow-ups on the results of cardiac procedures among the elderly, as well as investigations of cellular damage and subsequent recovery from ischemia (an organ's loss of arterial perfusion).

Aside from their inherent interest, the surgical research projects, along with the research programs touted at the

TCT2006 conference, are a window into the profound underlying forces driving the steady expansion of the health care sector. Looking beyond the plight of the CABG-dependent community cardiac surgeon, the field as a whole is moving very rapidly—new procedures, new devices, and expanding treatment possibilities for more and more conditions. I will touch on some of the policy implications of those in the next chapter, but in the rest of this one, I want to look briefly at what has been called the medical-industrial complex.

Money, Ethics, and Progress

George Bernard Shaw may not have been the first skeptic of the consequences of applying market principles to the practice of medicine, but he is among the more acerbic. From the preface to his play *The Doctor's Dilemma*:

> That any sane nation, having observed that you could provide for the supply of bread by giving bakers a pecuniary interest in baking for you, should go on to give surgeons a pecuniary interest in cutting off your leg, is enough to make one despair of political humanity.

Shaw penned those words a century ago, and he would have been dumbfounded at the commercialization of modern medicine. Ethical challenges can no longer be disposed of with a quip.

Pharmaceutical companies have been the primary villains in the ethical headlines of the past few years, often with good reason (Chapter 7). The apparently widespread practice of companies directly compensating, or otherwise rewarding, physicians for prescribing specific medications is offensive. Serving on a pharmaceutical company's speakers' bureau poses subtler questions. If you provide a direct service to a company, it's reasonable to be paid. And your audiences are typically medical professionals who know you're being paid and can weigh the facts for themselves. Questions revolve around whether you're being paid so much that it will influence your judgment. Allan Stewart told me that Bayer invited him to join their speakers' bureau. He gave it some thought, but decided to pass. "I use aprotinin in my surgery," he said, "but I don't think it's right for everyone. But I wouldn't feel right taking a lot of money from Bayer and telling people where they shouldn't use it."*

All doctors concede the ubiquity of ethical conflicts, while few admit to falling into them. But the data are not heartening. As we've seen, the supposedly independent physicians running company-sponsored drug trials are much more likely to reach favorable results than physicians running government or foundation-sponsored trials.

---

*In the framework of a widely used medical ethics textbook, Stewart described a conflict of *obligations*, the obligation to give value to his sponsor and to give the best information to his audience. Conflicts of obligations are almost inescapable—doctors' financial obligations to their employers often conflict with their obligations to their patients. Ethical conflicts arise when an obligation is transposed into a *self-interest*, like making money or advancing academically. Since Stewart expected that Bayer would not be happy if he shared his unvarnished views of aprotinin, he anticipated being caught in a conflict of interests and was right to turn down the opportunity.

Similarly, when physicians have a financial interest in a diagnostic imaging service, they are up to *four and a half times* more likely to refer patients for procedures than physicians who don't have such an interest. Money matters. Spinal fusion surgery is among the more rapidly growing procedures in recent years, and a number of the hardware companies have apparently made a concerted effort to recruit spinal surgeons as investors. Ethicists worry that the companies are intentionally creating conflicts of interest—creating extra incentives for surgeons both to recommend the surgery and to use specific hardware.

Ethical entwinements are especially complex in the development of medical devices and tools. Unlike a drug, the efficacy of a tool is hard to separate from the skill of the practitioner. Alain Cribier's first successful placements of what's become the Cribier-Edwards valve used a different access approach from that of the Jeff Moses / Marty Leon team at Columbia-Presbyterian. Moses and Leon are known as gifted interventionalists, but "Alain is extraordinary," Leon said, and they found his methods much too difficult to be applied safely. Adjusting a procedure, however, usually entails modifying the device, and that requires constant interaction between the company and the trial teams in an iterative process of trial and error. The newest versions of the Cribier-Edwards valve, for example, are smaller and have a more streamlined, lubricated, payload to overcome some of the difficulties encountered in the early rounds of trials.

Much of the interaction is informal. People like Felicia Brodzky, the da Vinci account rep I met in the OR (Chapter 8) are a key source of feedback. Brodzky probably sees a dozen operations a week, is in constant dialog with surgeons, and can bounce her impressions off experts like Argenziano. Each subgroup within the cardiothoracic division is a separate market. In late fall, I sat in on an inservice program for the perfusionists on a new-model percutaneous circulatory support machine. The demonstrator was a typically bright, technically aware, young company rep named Sherry Chang, and the session was clearly part of an ongoing conversation. Over the half hour or so that I watched, the team was full of suggestions for design tweaks, and at one point, Linda Mongero, the perfusionist director, asked Chang about a specific feature they had asked for in the past. Chang assured her that it was in development and might make the next release.

Academic medical centers frequently bring new device concepts to a near-end-product stage, which they rarely do in drugs. The MRI machine, fiberoptic endoscopes, laparascopic surgical tools, and the coronary angioplasty catheter are all blockbuster examples of devices developed in universities. But it still takes an industrial company to turn a working prototype into a marketable product—one that is reliable, incorporates relatively state-of-the-art component technologies, and can be sold at a reasonable price—and then to invest in operator training, usability improvement, and exploration of additional applications. The commercial development phase, however, usually goes much more smoothly if the academic inventors stay closely involved.

Faculty inventions are normally licensed through a university patent office and can involve serious money. After early-1980s congressional actions encouraged universities to exploit their intellectual property, Columbia's patent and licensing income soared from a half million dollars in 1985 to $32 million in 1995, and $160 million in 2005, tops among American universities. The inventors get a split of the fees, as agreed on a case-by-case basis. On the other hand, the vast majority of patents produce no income at all, while a small number of blockbusters typically account for almost all the earnings. Available data also suggest that biomedical patents are the most lucrative. In Columbia's 2005 report, seven of ten featured patents were in biomedicine. Many university patent offices never break even.

Most of the doctors have patent books, but more as a matter of principle, it seems, than in expectation of becoming rich. Allan Stewart told me that when he was an LVAD fellow, one of the companies invited him in for a product review. "I had a nice lunch," he said, "and gave them about six good ideas to improve the product. A little while later, they rolled out a new model that incorporated all of my ideas!" He grinned, "I thought they'd at least name a cannula after me. I told Mehmet about it," he went on, "and he said, 'Well, now you've learned your first lesson.' " Craig Smith has a number of patents but he has never earned any royalties, although one patent did get to the point of a company formation. Argenziano's A-rod device may be typical of most new medical tools. It's quite useful, but the market is small. The university didn't feel that it would justify the expense of filing a patent, so it was licensed to a private company in return for some divisional research support.

Annetine Gelijns, the codirector of InCHOIR (International Center for Health Outcomes and Innovation Research) at Columbia has thought as much and as well as anyone about the medical university–industry–government interaction. Academic physicians are supposed to contribute to advances in their specialties, she points out, and it is almost impossible to do that without participating in a complex matrix of academic, government, and industry exchanges. Gelijns hopes that the well-warranted concern over ethical risks doesn't obscure the importance of ensuring that the relationships actually generate a real stream of improvements in health care. At bottom, the question is whether there are practical frameworks that can improve transparency, promote a high rate of innovation, ensure reasonable fairness of financial outcomes, and still keep faith with the canons of medical ethics. That is a tall order, but the breakneck evolution of the industry over the past thirty or forty years makes it all the more pressing.

And finally, it is that same breakneck evolution that is at the root of the most pressing national policy question of all—how far can the country afford to expand its health care sector? Three developments, just from the cardiovascular arena, exemplify the challenge. If stents can safely produce results roughly equivalent to the CABG, and far less invasively, that is unalloyed progress. But the number of people who will receive stents—precisely because they are cheaper and less invasive—will be much larger than those who otherwise would have had CABGs. That will still be true even if there is a cutback on the use of the current models of drug-eluting stents.

Much the same could be said about the Cribier-Edwards valve, or about the evolving LVAD market.

Because of the terrific invasiveness of conventional valve surgery, a third to a half of patients who need valves are deemed unsuitable for the operation or refuse to undergo it. A much-less-invasive solution, in short, would sharply increase the number of valve interventions. So-called destination LVADs—LVADs to support people who are not eligible for a transplant because they are too old or too ill—are crushingly expensive, and have limited lives, so they are used mostly in experiments involving the sickest patients. But when LVADs become safe, highly functional, and at least as long-lived as transplants, as they almost certainly will in the not-distant future, a whole new market will emerge—moderately healthy people in the early stages of heart failure who could never be accommodated by the transplant lists. And as LVADs continue to improve, and eventually become full-replacement hearts, the bigger that market will get.

The list of new product opportunities, just in the cardiovascular field, could be multiplied almost endlessly. Half of all cardiac fatalities, for example, come without any warning to people who have no idea they have heart trouble. A major culprit may be "vulnerable plaque"— layers of occlusive material that are not obstructive enough to cause discomfort, or even to show up on an angiogram, but which can be easily fractured, releasing a sudden surge of debris which, if it collects at an arterial branchpoint or other structure, can cause a fatal blockage. One line of attack involves extremely precise imaging of the heart's internals, with MRIs, PET scans, CAT scans, and other technologies. Big companies—the GEs and the Siemenses of the world—are sniffing revenue bonanzas.

Automobiles were a hobbyist's industry until Henry Ford created the first inexpensive, high-function car. When desktop computers cost $10,000 and were very difficult to use, the only customers were monied geeks. Now that computers are much cheaper, much more useful, and easier to master, world spending runs in the half-trillion-dollar range.

The same iron laws apply to health care. Cheaper, better products *always* increase spending, and the faster the pace of improvement, the faster spending increases. That momentum is the primary driver of the headlong expansion of the health care sector. Ugly policy dilemmas have been looming for many years and can't be ignored or papered over much longer.

Chapter 10

POLICY

SOME TIME WITHIN THE NEXT TWENTY YEARS OR so, health care spending could consume about 30 percent of American GDP, or roughly twice its current share. Analysts have long been raising alarm at that prospect, but rather in the manner of Mao's dogs barking after the passing wagon train. Health care's growth momentum is now so powerful that there is no possibility of its being reversed in the foreseeable future.

Nor is it obvious that we should want to slow health care's growth. We can well afford it, and its effects on American jobs and overseas deficits will be much more positive than those from buying more Asian-made iPods and plasma televisions. As I will show below, even at very modest levels of economic growth, we could double the resources going into health care and still spend more on houses, video games, and SUVs, although the rate of spending growth for such items would slow.

To say that we can *afford* to ratchet up the rate of

health care spending, however, doesn't answer the question of how we're going to finance it. Under the pressures of global competition, the traditional American method of paying for health care as part of the employment benefit package has been visibly breaking down, and tens of millions of working families now have no coverage at all.

No one can predict the final shape of a new American health care financing dispensation, but the alignment of interests is such that one is virtually certain to emerge. Health care is now the country's largest private sector industry, and comprises much more than drug companies and hospital chains. American business icons like GE, IBM, 3M, Hewlett-Packard, and Intel are all making major bets on health care, and health care and biotechnology are among the hottest of targets for venture capital investors. Beyond that, the entire business community has an interest in better health care financing solutions, as both Ford's chairman, William Clay Ford, Jr., and Starbuck's CEO, Howard Schultz, have recently made clear. Congress, moreover, loves health care and has been singlemindedly pushing its expansion for more than sixty years. The most conservative, antientitlement administration and Congress in decades took control of the government in 2001; through 2006, its only significant health care initiative has been a major *increase* in Medicare benefits that was heavily lobbied by the pharmaceutical industry. In another striking demonstration of the clout of the medical-industrial complex, in 2002 Medicare approved final reimbursement rules for the drug-eluting stent a full nine months before the FDA even approved its use.

There are still reasons to worry about continued rapid

expansion of the health care sector. Its extraordinary technical achievements are among the nation's glories—we've seen some of them in this book. But operationally, the system is an expensive, paper-laden mess. Worse, our priorities appear hopelessly skewed toward the high-tech, high-glamour treatment sectors to the detriment of the important, dull parts—like prenatal care, childhood vaccinations, access to family doctors, and, for the chronically ill, tracking compliance with treatment regimens that prevent catastrophic flare-ups. In short, it's not the economic and financial implications of health care's growth that are troublesome, but the danger that rapid growth will make the current snarls even more intractable.

In the remainder of this chapter, I will first look at the forces driving health care's expansion and the implications for the national economy. Then I will summarize what I think are some of the most important managerial and policy challenges, and conclude with some speculations on potential financing solutions.

The Health Care Imperative

Few people seem to realize what a dynamic sector of the American economy health care has become. Companies like GE Healthcare (imaging, diagnostics, pharmaceutical manufacturing systems, patient monitoring systems, 45,000 employees, $15 billion in sales) are world leaders. Health care is an important driver of advances in electronics and biotechnology, is not especially susceptible to outsourcing, and is a positive offset to America's international fiscal deficits. It is also a generally good employer that pays above-average wages. The perfusionists at Columbia-Presbyterian are just one example of the burgeoning new professional and semiprofessional careers in health care, which include physicians' and surgeons' assistants, many varieties of imaging technicians, inhalation therapists, physical therapists, nurse-anesthestists, dental hygienists, and many, many more. One sign of the times: some of the deepest coverage of the late-2006 flap over possible complications from drug-eluting stents was in the *business* press rather than the science and health sections.

Despite the lamentations over "rising health care costs," procedure by procedure, technological advances are generally *reducing* costs, often by quite striking amounts, while bringing very large benefits in terms of extended, active, life spans. The very sharp drop in the death rate from heart attacks, for example, is substantially attributable to improvements in the technology of cardiac interventions. Modern pharmaceuticals are making major inroads in the treatment of depression, hypertension, diabetes, arthritis, and other chronic diseases, as well as steady advances against cancer. Surgical interventions to remove cataracts, or to replace hips, knees, or eye and ear parts, help people stay active and live longer. At the same time, laparoscopic and other microsurgical techniques make interventions cheaper, quicker, safer, and shorten recovery times. MRIs have replaced older invasive, often dangerous, diagnostic procedures, while advanced PET- and CAT-scanning systems facilitate far more informed interventions against cancers and heart and brain disease.

Just as in other markets, however, better, cheaper health

care products almost always *increase* total spending. Most gall bladder surgery, for example, is now performed on an outpatient basis: it's cheaper, requires minimal incisions, and gets you back to work sooner. Doctors are therefore more apt to recommend it, so total gall bladder spending is now higher than with the old, "expensive," full-surgery, inpatient methods. That same cycle whereby lower prices and better results increase spending can be seen in a long list of other standard therapies—cataract surgery is now a simple outpatient procedure that costs a fraction of what it used to, so millions of Americans have had it. Hip operations are surer, safer, with rapidly improving recovery times, so they are almost a *rite de passage* for senior golfers. LVADs and other heart-assist devices will soon be moving along a similar path.

The hard truth about health care is that death is usually the lowest-cost outcome. Twenty years or so ago, people in their seventies and above were considered too old for heart surgery; now they make up most of the patients, with very high success rates. Similarly, the raw number of annual deaths from cancer has been falling in the United States, even as the vulnerable population increases apace. But every victory that health care wins over traditional killers like heart disease and cancer preserves its best customers, and leads to years of more spending. The quickest way to reduce future Medicare costs would be to induce a lot more Americans to take up heavy smoking.*

---

*The macabre joke underlying the government's successful multibillion-dollar lawsuit against the tobacco companies, ostensibly to recover the excess health care costs of smokers, was that neither side could admit that smokers' high death rates saved the government

That steady expansion of health care's share of national spending, however, is quite consistent with the large sectoral shifts that have been a continuing feature of American growth. In the nineteenth century, most Americans worked on farms, compared to only about 2 percent today, although we produce and eat far more food. Fifty years ago, about a third of all workers were employed in manufacturing, compared to only 10 percent now, but the United States is still the world leader in real manufacturing output, and far ahead of China, which has six times as many manufacturing workers. Economic theory, in fact, suggests that health care *should* be expanding rapidly. The richer you get, the more you are likely to favor life-extending spending over additional consumption. The extra enjoyment from one more toy, in other words, can't begin to match up against an extra year of life to enjoy all of your toys.

But what about affordability? Could we really double health care's share of national product over the next twenty years without crippling the rest of the economy? That would depend on how fast the overall economy was growing. Consider three cases with twenty-year growth rates of 3 percent, 2 percent, and 1 percent annually after

---

money. Health care economists often try to offset the costs of medical interventions by the economic benefits of extended lives—if, say, an extra year of a "quality-adjusted" life is worth $100,000 (a common low-end assumption), a $300,000 heart transplant that extends life by ten years, on average, is well worth it. I've never found such arguments especially convincing. In real life cost-benefit analyses, the benefits are usually paid into the same coffers that the costs come from. But the assumed returns from Grandma's extra years of life are priced in theoretical dollars that you can't find on anyone's income statement.

inflation. At the 3 percent growth rate, health care would have to grow at 6.6 percent a year, about its current rate, to double its overall share, while the growth rate for everything else would be limited to about 2 percent. (Within that 2 percent, of course, some sectors would be declining rapidly, while some others would probably grow even faster than health care.) But if overall economic growth was only 2 percent per year, and health care doubled its share, the rest of the economy could grow at a rate of only 1 percent. And if the overall growth rate dropped to only 1 percent a year, the rest of the economy would need to stay essentially flat to accommodate health care's doubling.

Is it reasonable to expect the economy to grow at a 2 or 3 percent rate for the next twenty years? We can look at the record. Since 1929, there have been 67 ten-year periods* and 57 twenty-year periods. The average growth rate of the ten-year periods is 3.9 percent, and only one of the 67 was below 1 percent (1929–1939 tolled in at a dismal 0.9 percent). One other was 1.3 percent, nine others were between 2 and 3 percent, and the remaining 56 were all over 3 percent. Of the 57 twenty-year periods, only five came in below 3 percent, with the lowest at 2.2 percent. The average of all 57 was 3.7 percent. A 2 or 3 percent growth-rate assumption for the next twenty years is therefore well below the trend line. But even at those growth rates, health care could double its share of the economy and still allow continued growth in everything else.

*The 67 ten-year periods since 1929 comprise the sequence, 1929–1939, 1930–1940, 1931–1941 . . . 1995–2005.

Continued rapid growth in the health care sector, in short, would not only be economically affordable, but arguably a very positive development. It is an important driver of the high-technology industries that play to U.S. strengths. It is a good employer with multiple career ladders, and is pouring out an almost endless stream of new products and technologies that *work* and which people badly want. And to top it off, the spending mostly stays at home. That is a lot to like.

But there is another side to the story.

Health Care's Operational Tangle

The splendid American silos of excellence in cardiology and cardiac surgery, cancer treatment, and spine and brain disorders unfortunately operate in a world apart from the disgraceful mess on the ground. Consider a few recent research highlights. A high percentage of hospital discharge tests either never get to, or are never read by, the treating physician. There is only a weak correlation between a doctor's confidence in a diagnosis and its accuracy. A large number of physicians either aren't aware of, don't agree with, or don't follow currently accepted best practices in their specialties. Most physicians admit to little or no interest in quality control techniques. Only about a third have access to quality control data on their own practices or on the specialists they send patients to.

Despite spending, on average, about twice as much per capita as other industrialized countries, American primary care doctors are the least likely to have electronic record-keeping systems, and among the least likely to be able to order a prescription electronically or to access a patient's test results or hospital records. American doctors are also two to three times more likely to repeat a test because they can't get access to the previous test's results. On average, only half of Americans hospitalized for heart failure get written discharge instructions. And compared to patients in other countries, Americans are the most likely to use emergency rooms because they can't reach their usual doctor, and if they have a chronic disease, they are among the least likely to receive disease management oversight.

Most health care resources are consumed by a relatively small number of patients with one or more chronic diseases—heart disease, cancer, depression, diabetes, arthritis, or cognitive disorders. About a fifth of Medicare patients have five such disorders and, on average, have *fourteen* different physicians. Medicare itself concedes that it provides neither incentives nor facilities for coordinating interspecialty services. One study of American cardiac patients not only found very wide cost and quality gaps among different regions of the country, but also found that the regions with more slowly rising costs had fewer physicians per case, and better adherence to case management and follow-up protocols. That makes sense. Good case management and stable physician oversight means fewer big-ticket crisis interventions. Confusion costs.

Well-intended attempts to "improve coordination" or "realign incentives" may just make things worse. Bureaucratic paper processing, much of it related to reimbursement systems, already consumes as much as 20 percent of all health care resources. Payment systems are also shot through with perversities. The primary care physicians, the front-line docs who are supposed to shepherd their patients through the copious wonders of modern medicine, have been among the hardest hit by the compression of medical fees over the past decade or so. The standard ten- or fifteen-minute office visit may be enough for healthy people, but it can't begin to get the job done for the chronically ill, who tend to bounce from specialist to specialist pretty much on their own.

Payment systems also tend to reward procedures. Cardiology became a much more lucrative profession once cardiologists went into the angioplasty and stent business. Oncologists can make large profits on the difference between Medicare chemotherapy drug payment rates and their actual costs, and there is evidence that the size of the profit opportunity may affect the choice of drug. Dermatology, with its huge kit of office-based procedures, is reputedly one of the most lucrative of the medical professions.

TMR, or transmyocardial revascularization, is a good example of the procedure as money-spinner. It is a method of improving coronary perfusion by using lasers to burn microscopic channels in heart muscle. Much of the development was done at Columbia-Presbyterian; Craig Smith filed some of the early patents. TMR was approved by the FDA in 1998 based on clinical trials in which treated patients reported relief of angina pain, even though the mechanism of action was unclear.* The procedure is

---

*The original idea was that the new channels would increase blood flow, but autopsy evidence suggested that the channels mostly closed up. An FDA review speculated that the injury to the muscle tissue stimulated angiogenesis (new vessel growth), or that it may have

almost never used at Columbia-Presbyterian, however, because Smith and his colleagues are convinced that the positive trial results are classic subjective, placebo-effectlike phenomena. But since TMR has been approved by the FDA, almost all medical plans will pay for it, and fee-hungry cardiac surgeons are enthusiastically adopting it in their practices.

The defects of American health care are the flip side of its virtues. The deep commitment to technological innovation, the penchant for rich and complex service arrays, the ease with which patients can shop among specialists and treatment options, are all unique, and have generated an extraordinary record of accomplishment in cutting-edge medicine. But along with that comes a free-wheeling approach to the introduction of new, often unproven technologies, hit-or-miss coordination of services, and very high costs—at least 25 percent higher than in any other industrialized country. It is a system that seems designed for the affluent, educated patient with the most comprehensive insurance coverage. But for the working stiff with minimum coverage it can be confusing, difficult to access, and possibly even dangerous.

The fascination with cutting-edge technologies is evident in the government's research priorities. Half of the federal basic and applied research budget goes to health care, far more than to any other function. The director of

---

destroyed nerves that were sensitive to pain, or that, since the end point was essentially subjective—rate your pain on a scale—and it's hard to blind surgical interventions, the reported improvements may have been mostly a placebo effect.

the National Institutes of Health recently estimated total federal health care research outlays over the past thirty years at nearly $400 billion, more than $30 billion of which went to cardiovascular research. Current research priorities are decidedly forward-looking—breakthroughs in genomics, in microsurgery, in new classes of pharmaceuticals, all of which may someday feed into blockbuster new products for drug and medical device companies. And consider the spectacle of states, with generally poor records in vaccinations and child and maternal health programs, competing with each other to mount multibillion-dollar stem cell research programs.

In such an environment, it should be no surprise that the United States has such a high-cost health care system. American payers, including Medicare, pretty much pay for any treatment that has been approved by the FDA, or is otherwise part of standard medicine, leaving the question of appropriateness up to the individual doctor. A senior executive at Guidant, one of the leading competitors in stents, said that in Europe, "when a new therapy is trying to find a reimbursement budget, the money has to come from other therapies. . . . So it's a very slow process. We know that innovative devices do get accepted, but it's done at a very slow rate." America, by contrast, is the device maker's dream market, and the pace of adoption of drug-eluting stents (DES) has been almost frenzied. In just a couple of years, the total number of stents placed roughly doubled, with almost all of them the more expensive DES versions. By 2005, American usage of DES was more than twice that in the advanced countries of Europe. Safe use of DES, however, requires prolonged anticlotting medica-

tions, usually both aspirin and Plavix, an expensive drug.*
The explosion in DES placement also means that many
more heart surgery patients have been on prolonged anticlotting therapies, which has been a major factor in the
increased use of aprotinin in heart surgery. And so the
expense impact ripples on.

The recent—and still inconclusive—revelations of
possible long-term problems with DES, however, suggest
that explosive growth may not always be in the best interest of patients. And it is interesting that European cardiologists, who were more cautious in adopting DES in the
first place, have been much quicker than Americans to pull
back. In the wake of suggestions at a late-2006 FDA advisory committee hearing that DES may be inappropriate
for many current patients, the business press was quick to
reassure investors that the effect on American practice
would be small. In my own unscientific sample of a half-
dozen Web-based continuing medical education programs
on DES in the wake of the FDA meeting (on Web pages
festooned with the logos of stent makers), the consistent
advice seemed to be "don't change current practice." (In

---

*An important subsidiary question is whether patients actually stick
with the anticlotting regimens. Anecdotal evidence, at least, suggests
that depending on their insurance, many probably don't, which is
dangerous. The rights to Plavix (clopidogrel) are owned by Sanofi-
Aventis (in Europe) and Bristol-Myers Squibb (BMS). As of early
2007, there is a complicated patent dispute between BMS and several generic drug makers as to whether the clopidogrel patents expired
in 2003, or are good until 2011, as BMS maintains. In addition,
Sanofi-Aventis and BMS are under investigation for possible antitrust
violations for attempting to forestall potential generic competition.
Annual sales of Plavix exceed $6 billion.

a spring 2007 presentation, however, Marty Leon specifically endorsed a pullback in DES usage, in part because of the dangers of prolonging antiplatelet therapy to prevent clotting events.) The same kind of frenzied proliferation was seen during the explosive growth phase of CABG surgery forty years ago, and of laparascopic surgery twenty years ago. Over the longer haul, both made substantial contributions to the health of Americans, but few would dispute that the breakneck pace of the rollouts quickly outstripped the capabilities of physicians, or the understanding of the procedures, and that many patients were placed in harm's way as a consequence.

A distinguishing feature of the current era, however, is that as the cornucopia of available treatments keeps expanding, the high-cost, leading-edge-only, American style of care delivery is becoming unaffordable even for the strongest companies. The first reaction, in the 1990s, was to slow cost growth by clogging the system with paperwork—HMO horror stories became staple fare for late-night television comics. More recently, companies have been shedding costs by shifting them to workers, outsourcing functions to lower-cost vendors with limited benefits, or simply eliminating the health care benefit altogether.

The result is a dreadful muddle—swamps of paperwork, spotty coverage for almost everyone but the higher-strata employees at the larger companies, growing numbers of working people with no coverage at all, and an ever-richer and more complex array of services that is difficult even for healthy people to navigate on their own, much less the old and chronically ill.

The paperwork morass is aggravated by the strange proclivity of American analysts and pundits to focus almost exclusively on the payment system as the agent of change. David Cutler, one of the finest of American health care economists, in discussing the gaping regional differences in American care proposes to solve the problem by "experiments with financial incentives" for both patients and providers. And the economist and *New York Times* columnist David Leonhardt, after reviewing evidence of overuse of stents, concluded that "sometimes, Medicare or an insurance policy should nudge people away from the latest, greatest treatment." Sounds simple, right? Use your payment power to "nudge" people in the right direction. Now imagine trying to draft the payment regulations and supporting documentation required to do that. And also consider how irrelevant all the multiple payment systems are in determining how the surgeons at Columbia Presbyterian run their practices (see Chapter 9). I don't mean to single out Cutler and Leonhardt, for dozens and dozens of policy articles take a similar line. But a little common sense should suggest that payment systems are hopelessly blunt tools, and any attempts to fine-tune them to drive specific behavior is likely to end in yet more muddle.*

---

*As this is written, there is great enthusiasm for "pay for performance," or P4P, systems. There are in fact some protocols so widely accepted—almost all cardiac patients should be on aspirin regimens—that it makes sense to penalize or reward practices for their compliance. But the number of instances where such rules can be definitively enforced, relative to the totality of health care services, will be very small. To speak of P4P as a major step toward higher quality and less expensive health care strikes me as a counsel of desperation.

The Kaiser-Permanente programs are one of the few American health care systems that do a reasonably good job of maintaining high-quality practice standards while resisting the introduction of new technologies of dubious benefit. But they don't do it with payment tweaks; instead, they establish and enforce explicit practice rules. If the internal practice-standard committees are not convinced of the value of TMR, say, then plan physicians may not use it. And if the committees deem that 90 percent beta-blocker compliance should be standard for cardiac patients, they have the clout to enforce it. The distinguishing feature of the Kaiser-Permanente plans, however, is that there is a *medical management* layer. Doctors are supervising other doctors to ensure that they are providing treatment in accord with agreed standards. The cherished myth of the American independent practitioner is that every doctor keeps up with best practices all by herself. But as the survey data cited earlier suggest, it is a myth—a myth on the same scale as the hopelessly doomed notion that one can somehow create good medical management by fine-tuning payment systems.

Can We Do Better?

The American political process, unlike some European parliamentary systems, is built to resist sweeping change. Although basic interest alignments are pointing toward a major reorganization of American health care, it is likely to happen incrementally and take a long time. Liberals should stop hoping for radical change, like a shift to the

Canadian "single-payer" model of health insurance, while conservatives should drop favorite fetishes, like that of a "private-sector" health care system, which is already a fiction. More than half of all health care costs are now paid by the government, and demographic and technological trends are likely to push that number into the two-thirds range within the foreseeable future.

What follows is a not a set of recommendations, but a rough forecast of what I think is likely to evolve from a rolling series of health care minicrises over the next couple of decades:

+ The federal government will establish a minimum standard Basic Health Plan. Offering the plan would be mandatory for all employers above a very low minimum size. The Basic Plan would also replace Medicaid and Medicare.
+ All qualified insurance vendors could market and service the plans. They would compete on price and service rather than on the benefit provisions.*

---

*There is a direct, and successful, precedent on this point. In the 1970s, so-called Medigap insurance programs to supplement Medicare coverage sprang up by the thousands. Provisions were so complicated that even the most capable seniors had difficulty choosing among plans and frequently found themselves overcharged. Congress stepped in in 1981 and mandated ten basic plans. All Medigap vendors had to market all ten plans, and benefit provision had to be identical from vendor to vendor. The market quickly stabilized around three or four of the plans, companies competed hard on price and service quality, and the vast majority of seniors purchased the coverage. It is a pity that a similar approach was not used for the new Medicare Part D pharmaceutical plan.

- Limits on both covered procedures and treatment costs would be maintained by a system of national and regional committees comprising medical, financial, and business representation. Copays, deductibles, and similar devices would be applied to ensure efficient use of resources.

- No doctors would be obligated to participate in the plan. But those who wish to do so would join one or more physician networks; would agree to comprehensive data exchange, electronic record-keeping, and similar standards; and would comply with protocol- and quality-oriented standards for chronic disease management, childhood health maintenance, and other treatment processes. All physician quality outcomes and protocol compliance would be tracked by network managers.

- The cost of coverage would be contributory for employers and employees subject to a wage-based sliding scale. Premiums for low-wage employees, the elderly, and the unemployed would be subsidized by the federal government. An employer's premium for the basic plan might also be capped (subsidized) to maintain competitiveness in a global marketplace.

- Insurance companies would be free to offer carriage-trade luxury plans for favored employee groups or supplemental coverage for Basic Plan enrollees. But only the Basic Plan payments would be tax-advantaged.

- Government subventions would be covered by a dedicated, progressive, broad-based tax. The program would therefore have substantial redistributive elements. Note, however, that virtually all tax proceeds would be immediately recycled into the private health care economy.

Some parallel developments that would also be helpful:

+ A substantial conversion of NIH and related federal research dollars from disease-focused research to the development of the data-mining technologies and quality protocols required for high-technology medicine.
+ Development of a cadre of medical managers to develop and maintain quality systems. Managerial overhead may possibly *increase*, but the dead weight of meaningless paper shuffling would be mostly eliminated, so the net effect may be small.
+ Development of much more powerful industry-government quality inspection and error-detection systems. It will be essential to replace the current medical malpractice system with a workmen's-compensationlike system based on expert inquiry.
+ A system of industry-government review panels to monitor current therapies and technologies, establish allowability within the Basic Plan, and maintain best-practice protocols.

The proposals above are merely suggestive, and the universe of reasonable variations is very large. And it will take a long time: the near-term possibility of comprehensive restructuring is probably close to nil. But thorough-going reform will come, because, quite separately from its glorious technologies, American health care is careening toward a slow-motion political and administrative debacle, and too many powerful economic stakeholders have too much at risk to allow that to happen.

Appendix I

HOW THE HEART WORKS

Basic Structure. There are four main chambers and four main valves in the heart, two on each side.

The *right atrium* collects venous blood from the big pipeline called the vena cava. (The superior, or upper, end of the vena cava collects blood from the head and upper body, while the inferior, or lower, end of the vena cava collects blood from the lower body.)

When the heart is relaxed (diastole), blood flows from the vena cava into the right atrium. As pressure builds in the atrium, the *tricuspid valve* pops open, and the blood flows from the right atrium into the *right ventricle*.

As the right ventricle fills, the heart contracts (systole), and the pressure in the ventricle shuts the tricuspid valve and opens the *pulmonary valve*, so the blood flows into the pulmonary artery, which takes it to the lungs.

Four pulmonary veins, two from each lung, dump freshly oxygenated blood from the lungs into the *left atrium* when the heart is relaxed. As pressure builds in the

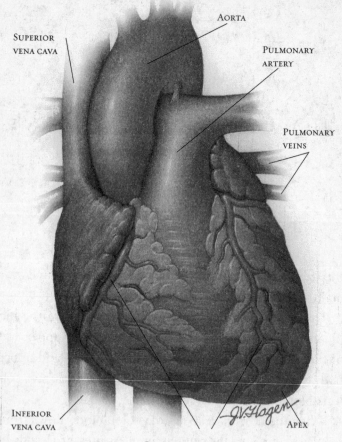

SUPERIOR
VENA CAVA

AORTA

PULMONARY
ARTERY

PULMONARY
VEINS

INFERIOR
VENA CAVA

APEX

CORONARY ARTERIES

left atrium, the *mitral valve* pops open, and blood flows from the left atrium into the *left ventricle*.

As the left ventricle fills, the heart contracts (systole) and the pressure in the ventricle shuts the mitral valve and opens the *aortic valve*, so the blood flows into the aorta and the body's arterial system.

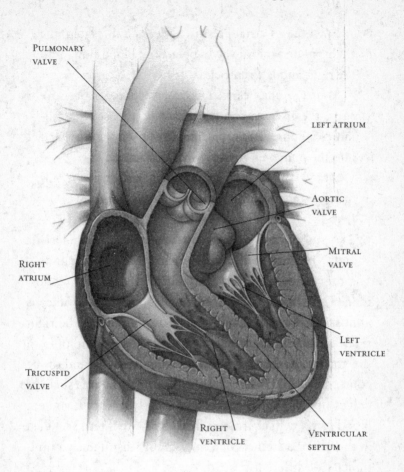

PULMONARY VALVE

LEFT ATRIUM

AORTIC VALVE

MITRAL VALVE

RIGHT ATRIUM

LEFT VENTRICLE

TRICUSPID VALVE

RIGHT VENTRICLE

VENTRICULAR SEPTUM

The right and left sides of the heart, of course, relax and contract in unison. The overall cycle can be divided into four phases:

STAGE 1. Heart is relaxed, all four valves are closed, and blood is flowing into both the right and left atria.

STAGE 2. As atrial pressure exceeds a threshold, the tricuspid and mitral valves open, and blood flows into the right and left ventricles.

STAGE 3. The heart contracts. Ventricular pressure rises, the tricuspid and mitral valves close, the pulmonary and aortic valves open, and blood is ejected into the pulmonary artery and the aorta.

STAGE 4. The ventricles begin relaxation and the pulmonary and aortic valves close.

The stages of the heart cycle generate characteristic sounds. In a healthy heart, there are two main sounds— "da-dum." The "da" is the sound of the mitral valve closing. (The tricuspid, which closes at the same time, is almost silent because of the lower pressures on the right side.) The second sound, the "dum," is the sound of both the aortic and pulmonary valves closing at the end of the contractile stage. Abnormalities in the heart, such as valves not opening or closing properly, create turbulent blood flows with characteristic sounds. An internist skilled in the use of a stethoscope can reliably distinguish a multiplicity of different heart diseases.

The Heartbeat. The myocardium, or the heart muscle, consists primarily of specialized muscle cells called cardiomyocytes. Each cell is of a roughly oblong shape and contains two parallel planes of different lengths that can slide past each other—call them Plane A and Plane B. Plane A also has a hooking apparatus that can engage with a binding site on Plane B.

When the cell is in its relaxed state, the binding site is blocked; the two planes are unconnected and have slid so that their opposite ends are as far apart as possible, stretching the cell to its maximum length.

When energy (from ATP, our cells' universal storage battery of chemoelectrical energy) is released, calcium ions flow into the cell. The calcium unblocks the binding site on Plane B. Plane A's hooking apparatus engages the binding site, and pulls Plane B backward along its length. The cell becomes shorter, and the heart contracts.

A feedback mechanism generates a second release of ATP-mediated energy, and the surrounding cell matrix reabsorbs the calcium. Plane B's binding site is blocked, the hooking apparatus disengages, and the cell relaxes and lengthens once more.

The ticktock extension and contraction of heart muscle as calcium ions move into and out of the cell is strikingly like that of the escapement mechanism in a spring-driven watch. And so long as there is a suitable supply of ATP-mediated energy, the cell will continue to expand and contract in a regular fashion for as long as it lives.

Heart Rhythm

Cardiomyocytes all beat, but an effective heart function requires that they beat in rhythm.

The heartbeat is controlled by the body's autonomic, or involuntary, nervous system. An island of cardiomyocytes located at the juncture of the vena cava and the right atrium pick up the signal from the nervous system and beat in unison. They are called the "SA node," although by themselves they are indistinguishable from other cardiomyocytes. A chemoelectrical signal ripples outward from the SA node through the rest of the heart and imposes an orderly beating rhythm. Since the radiation of the electrical signal through the heart takes time, the beat propagates throughout the heart in a measurable wave pattern. Better understanding of those patterns has been the basis of much recent progress in pacemakers.

The Coronary Arteries

The two main coronary arteries arise from the aorta just above the aortic valve. The left main coronary artery immediately divides into the left anterior descending artery, the "LAD" (it runs down the front of the left side of the heart), and the circumflex artery, which runs along the top of the heart to the back, with many downward branches. The right coronary artery supplies blood to the right side and lower reaches of the heart.

Corona is the Latin word for "crown." The coronary arteries' branching pattern around the top of the heart and down reminded early anatomists of a crown, hence the name.

Since the left ventricle is the workhorse of the heart—it has to move blood the greatest distance—blockages of the left main artery or of the LAD are usually the most life-threatening and are usually repaired with a CABG (coronary artery bypass graft) rather than a stent, for greater durability.

Some Factoids

The average adult has about five quarts of blood, and about 50,000 miles of blood vessels, the vast majority of them too small to see.

At rest, your entire volume of blood is circulated through your body about once every minute.

Total blood volume moved each day is about 1,800 gallons.

When necessary, your heart can increase the volume of circulation up to four to seven times the resting rate.

Over the course of a lifetime, the heart beats about 2.5 billion times and moves about 50 million gallons of blood.

THE NEW YORK STATE CARDIAC HOSPITAL RATING SYSTEM

The Rating System. New York State first adopted an aggressive regulatory posture toward cardiac surgery in the 1980s, a time when revenue-hungry hospitals were proliferating new heart surgery centers, and surgical mortality rates were rising sharply. Since there was good evidence that related high volumes to good outcomes, both for centers and surgeons, a new certification process focused on closing down low-volume centers and limiting the number of new ones coming on line.

To support its certification program, in 1989 the State created a system for tracking CABG outcomes, defined as risk-adjusted mortality rates, for both centers and individual surgeons. The system was extended to valves in 1998, but because of lower volumes, reported outcomes are in three-year moving averages, so the first valve report was issued only with the 2000 data.

The risk adjustment was based on a statistical model of

the entire State database that related mortality to objective case characteristics, like age, a reop, ejection fraction, renal failure, and the like. The hospitals rate their own cases, subject to selective State audits that concentrate on risk ratings that look too high. The ratings and rankings were originally supposed to be confidential, but they eventually became public, partly due to a Freedom of Information suit.

The system must be counted an almost unalloyed success, in great part due to the consistent, persistent management of Edward Hannan, a professor at the State University School of Public Health in Albany, who has been its primary designer and overseer since the beginning. It has been replicated in five other states as well as in a reporting network for hospitals in New England. All but two of the other networks also report their results publicly. A similar system was being debated in Great Britain as of March 2007.

The implementation of the report coincided with a sharp drop in New York State mortality rates. Using Medicare's risk-adjusted CABG outcome data, New York State's CABG mortality rate dropped 28 percent from 1989 to 1993, compared to 13 percent in the rest of the country. That advantage was maintained in subsequent years. In the 1994–1999 period, the last one for which Medicare data are available, New York State's CABG mortality rate averaged 67 percent of the nationwide rate, a statistically significant difference.

It's reasonable to believe that the reporting system has something to do with New York State's excellent performance. But it's harder to point to exactly why. It's certainly not, as free-market theorists hoped, because consumers shifted their business to hospitals with the best ratings, for low ratings had no effect on subsequent volumes. (And consumers don't choose their heart hospitals anyway; their cardiologists do.) Nor is there any support in the data for complaints from within the profession that ratings-wary surgeons were avoiding difficult cases, or referring them out of state. The most plausible, if probably not the entire, explanation is that published surgical ratings forced the worst performers out of the system, either through embarrassment or from quiet pressure from colleagues.

Columbia-Presbyterian and the Ratings. In Chapter 6, I recounted the sudden spike in Columbia-Presbyterian's one-year mortality rankings in 2001. They were reflected two years later in the statewide compilations, just at the time of the Clinton surgery, drawing much critical comment from the *New York Times*. It clearly did not have any affect on cardiologist referrals—as it probably shouldn't have—since it does appear to have been a one-year (actually, seven-month), so-far-unexplained blip.

But I found it interesting that Columbia-Presbyterian almost certainly *understates* their performance for State reporting purposes (although possible underscoring had little to do the 2001 results). I take that as another example of the academic mind-set; I can't believe that a for-profit hospital wouldn't pay very close attention to their numbers.

I show the CABG data from ten years of reports below. For a hospital, three different numbers are tracked. The first is the OMR, or observed (actual) mortality rate. The second is the EMR, or expected mortality rate, based on the State's risk-adjustment formula, and the third is RAMR, or risk-adjusted mortality rate. The hospital RAMR is then compared to the statewide mortality rate.*

The formula for a hospital's risk-adjusted mortality rate is OMR/EMR times the statewide mortality rate. For example, if the statewide rate is 4 deaths per 100 patients, the hospital's observed mortality rate is also 4, and its expected rate is 2, the formula produces (4/2) times 4 = 8. The hospital's risk-adjusted rate is twice as bad as the statewide average, reflecting the fact that its average case was only half as risky. On the other hand, if the hospital's expected mortality rate is high—assume it's 8, meaning it handles very difficult cases—then the formula would be (4/8) times 4 = 2: the hospital's risk-adjusted outcome now shows that its performance is twice as good as the statewide average, even though its observed mortality rate is the same.

Here are the ten-year data on Columbia-Presbyterian's CABG mortality.

	1995	1996	1997	1998	1999	2000	2001	2002	2003	2004
C-P Observed Mortlity Rate	1.89	1.74	2.14	1.67	2.35	2.04	3.70	1.92	0.73	1.72
C-P Expected Mortlity Rate	2.46	2.45	2.14	2.04	1.91	2.12	2.05	1.81	1.32	1.92
C-P Risk-adjusted Mortlity Rate	1.93	1.73	2.22	1.76	2.76	2.24	3.93	2.40	0.89	1.88
NYS Mortlity Rate	2.52	2.44	2.22	2.15	2.24	2.32	2.18	2.27	1.61	2.09
C-P Expected Rate – NYS Mortlity Rate	-0.06	0.01	-0.08	-0.11	-0.33	-0.20	-0.13	-0.46	-0.29	-0.17

*The formulas set the statewide actual, expected, and risk-adjusted mortality rates as identical.

In every year but two, Columbia-Presbyterian's observed mortality was lower than the state average. But in every year except 1996, the EMR, or the difficulty of Columbia-Presbyterian's cases, was also lower than the statewide average. In other words, Columbia-Presbyterian consistently rated itself as having easier cases than the state's other hospitals, thereby inflating its risk-adjusted mortality rate, in some years by a substantial amount. Even with the low EMRs, however, Columbia-Presbyterian risk-adjusted mortality rate exceeded the state rate only three times.

Columbia-Presbyterian's low-risk ratings do not seem plausible. The hospital, after all, is one where other hospitals send their hard cases, and the surgeons pride themselves, as Allan Stewart put it, in taking "the high-risk surgery, the case that's been turned down by two other surgeons." I looked closely at the data for 2003, which were released in 2005 when I was doing the research. In both CABGs and valves, Columbia-Presbyterian's case difficulty rating put it in the bottom quintile of all state hospitals. Interestingly, in CABGs, all three of its New York affiliates, including one that was in a start-up mode and had restrictions on the cases it could accept, had higher difficulty rankings than Columbia-Presbyterian did. When I ran those numbers by Ed Hannan, he asked "Why would they shoot themselves in the foot like that? We don't audit for *under*scoring." I have no explanations for the low-risk ratings, except as another example of academic behavior.

NOTES

Chapter 2: A VERY SHORT HISTORY OF HEART SURGERY

Stephen Westaby's masterful survey, *Landmarks in Cardiac Surgery* (Oxford, U.K.: Isis Medical Media, 2000) is a basic source. Westaby is himself a cardiovascular surgeon who has made a number of contributions to transplant and artificial heart technology, and is personally acquainted with almost all the great innovators in his narrative. For ancient roots, see *ibid.*, pp. 1–12. For theory of "humors, " see A. C. Crombie, *Augustine to Galileo* (London: Heineman, 1959), vol. 1, pp. 170–175. For two early surgeries, Westaby, *op. cit.*, p. 20. Phrase "negro cabin," is from the original case report. For World War I and intrawar years, *ibid.*, pp. 22–27. For growth of cardiac disease, see Jesse H. Ausubel et al., "Death and the Human Environment: the United States in the 20th Century," *Technology in Society* 23:2 (Spring 2001): 131–146. For the cardiopulmonary bypass machine, Westaby, *op. cit.*, pp. 51–52, 63; for valves, *ibid.*, 160–163; for pre-CABG coronary surgery and Favaloro, *ibid.*, pp. 188–198. Later-period CABG data are from Center for Disease Control, *National Hospital Discharge*

Survey, 2003, Table 100, released in 2005. The statistic "4 percent of CABG" is from Annetine Gelijns et al., "Evidence, Politics, and Technological Change," *Health Affairs* 24:1 (January–February 2005): 29–40, at 31–32. The statistics on the decline of heart attack death rates are from a table supplied to me by Thomas J. Thom, statistician, National Heart, Lung, and Blood Institute. The data on federal research spending is from *U.S. Budget, 2007: Analytical Perspectives*, p. 49, Table 5-1; cumulative health research spending is from Elias Zerhouni, "Testimony Before the Senate Subcommittee on Labor—HHS—Education Appropriations," May 19, 2006. (I converted Zerhouni's per capita numbers.)

Chapter 3: ARTISANS AT WORK

On the spread of minimally invasive surgical techniques in the 1990s, see Annetine Gelijns et al., "The Dynamics of Technological Change in Medicine," *Health Affairs* (Summer 1994), 28–46, at 40. The switch operation is just old enough for longer-term data to become available. One of the first reports was for "Fontan" kids—born with a single ventricle. The rebuilding required is very similar, however, so I think it's reasonable to extrapolate those data to the switch. See M. E. Mitchell et al., "Intermediate Outcomes After the Fontan Procedure in the Current Era," *Journal of Thoracic and Cardiovascular Surgery* 131:1 (January 2006): 172–180.

Chapter 4: THE MOST PRECIOUS RESOURCE

All transplant data in this chapter, including historical data, come from the comprehensive data sets maintained by the federal Organ Procurement and Transplant Network (OPTN), the supervising transplant agency. They are produced on a hospi-

tal, state, and national basis. The Web site is www.optn
.org/data/. The staff at the OPTN were also helpful in navigat-
ing and interpreting the data sets. The CIT data I cite are the
standard ones; recent data suggest that >300-minute CITs may
be tolerable with the most recent cardioprotective measures: F.
T. Mitropoulos et al., "Outcome of Hearts with Cold Ischemic
Time Greater than 300 Minutes," *European Journal of Cardiothoracic Surgery* 28 (July 2005): 143–145. The revised regulations are from Department of Health and Human Services, 42
CFR Part 121 Organ Procurement and Transplantation Network. The revised allocation criteria are in 121.8. For LVADs
and the future of the mechanical heart, see Mehmet C. Oz et
al., "Left Ventricular Assist Devices as Permanent Heart Failure Therapy: The Price of Progress," *Annals of Surgery* 238:4
(October 2003): 577–585; and Jonathan M. Chen et al., "The
Future of Left Ventricular Assist Device Therapy in Adults,"
Nature Clinical Practice 3:7 (July 2006): 346–347. The capsule
history is from Stephen Westaby, *Landmarks in Cardiac Surgery* (Oxford, U.K.: Isis Medical Media, 2000), pp. 287–296.

Chapter 5: ERIKA'S STORY

Erika suffered from a subspecies of cardiomyopathy called
"restrictive cardiomyopathy." For more detail, see the review
article Sudhir S. Kushwaha et al., "Restrictive Cardiomyopathy," *New England Journal of Medicine* 336:4 (January 23,
1997): 267–276.

Chapter 6: SCHOOL FOR HEART SURGEONS

Comments from Sherwin Nuland are from an interview. For the
residents' work limitations: IPRO, "Working Hours and Conditions Post-Graduate Trainees, Annual Compliance Assessment,

Contract Year 4, 10/1/04–9/30/05," available at www.ipro.org; and see Edward E. Whang et al., "Implementing Resident Work Hour Limitations: Lessons from the New York State Experience," *Obstetrical and Gynecological Survey* 58:8 (August 2003): 531–532, reporting a survey of resident attitudes. The majority agreed that it had improved their quality of life, while about half felt they were missing learning opportunities. Charles L. Bosk, *Forgive and Remember: Managing Medical Failure* (Chicago: University of Chicago Press, 1979) is a sociologist's account of a year's field research at a large academic general surgery program and concentrates on the M&M process. I came across it after I had been at Columbia-Presbyterian for some months and was struck by how much Bosk's experiences were like my own. Everyone seemed very skeptical of him when he first arrived, but once he had been somehow certified as a legitimate presence, no one withheld anything. The dynamic of decision-making was also much like the one I witnessed. The similarities are the more striking because Bosk's research took place more than twenty-five years ago. For "human factors" research, see Marc R. DeLeval et al., "Human Factors and Cardiac Surgery: A Multicenter Study," *Journal of Cardiovascular and Thoracic Surgery* 110:4 (April 2000): 661–672. For an example of airline studies, see Christopher D. Wickens et al., *Flight to the Future: Human Factors in Air Traffic Control* (Washington, D.C.: National Academies Press, 1997).

Chapter 7: THE MEASUREMENT PROBLEM

The aprotinin article is Dennis T. Mangano et al., "The Risk Associated with Aprotinin in Cardiac Surgery," *New England Journal of Medicine* 354:4 (January 26, 2006): 353–365. The "not prudent" quote is on p. 353. The Vioxx paper mentioned by Shanewise is C. Bombardier et al., "Comparison of Upper Gastrointestinal Toxicity of Rofecoxib and Naproxen in

Patients with Rheumatoid Arthritis," *New England Journal of Medicine* 343:21 (November 23, 2000): 1520–1528. The other study mentioned in the note is Keyvan Karkouti et al., "A Propensity Score Case-Control Comparison of Aprotinin and Tranexamic Acid in High-Transfusion-Risk Cardiac Surgery," *Transfusion* 46:3 (January 20, 2006): 327–338. The meta-analyses supporting Bayer include: D. A. Henry et al., "Anti-fibrinolytic Use for Minimisimg Perioperative Allogeneic Blood Transfusion" (Review), *Cochrane Database of Systematic Reviews*, 2006, 1–114 (first published on-line in October 25, 1999. The Cochrane publication lists sixty-one randomized clinical trials of aprotinin, but because of data-comparison issues, the meta-analysis draws from only twenty-nine. Probably the second-most-often-cited meta-analysis is A. Sedrakyan et al., "Effect of Aprotinin on Clinical Outcomes in Coronary Artery Bypass Graft Surgery: A Systematic Review and Meta-Analysis of Randomized Clinical Trials," *Journal of Thoracic and Cardiovascular Surgery* 128:3 (September 2004): 442–448. I also had several email exchanges with Dr. Tom Treasure, one of the authors of the Sedrakyan paper.

The Problem with Drug Companies

Aprotinin sales data are from the company's "Bayer R&D, Investor Day 2005," December 8, 2005, London. Sales were reported in euros, which I converted at a 1.25 dollar:euro ratio. On drug prices in America, see Patricia Danzon et al., "Prices and Availability of Pharmaceuticals: Evidence from Nine Countries," *Health Affairs* (Web exclusive, October 29, 2003), W3-521–536. For the drug company contribution to drug development, see Annetine C. Gelijns, *Innovations in Clinical Practice: The Dynamics of Medical Technology Development* (Washington, D.C.: National Academy Press, 1991), pp. 40–61, 105–123.

For a comprehensive denunciation of current drug company practice, see Marcia Angell, *The Truth About Drug Companies: How They Deceive Us and What to Do About It*, rev. ed.

(New York: Random House, 2005), and Jerome P. Kassirer, *On The Take: How Medicine's Complicity with Big Business Can Endanger Your Health* (New York: Oxford University Press, 2005). Angell and Kassirer were successive editors of the *New England Journal of Medicine*, and so had a good window into drug company trial management and publication practices. For Big Pharma lobbying, see Angell, *op. cit.*, pp. 198–199, 214–216; and for conflicts of members of FDA advisory committees, *ibid.*, pp. 210–211. The prohibition on the Stanford doctors is from "Stanford Won't Let Doctors Accept Gifts," AP, September 12, 2006, *MSNBC*. For financial settlements: "TAP Pharmaceutical Products, Inc., and Seven Others Charged with Health Care Crimes: Company Agrees to Pay $875 Million to Settle Charges," DOJ press release, October 3, 2001; "Astrazeneca Pharmaceuticals LP Pleads Guilty to Healthcare Crime: Company Agrees to Pay $355 Million to Settle Charges," DOJ press release, June 20, 2003; "Warner-Lambert to Pay $430 Million to Resolve Criminal and Civil Health Care Liability Relating to Off-Label Promotion," DOJ press release, May 13, 2004. Warner-Lambert was purchased by Pfizer in 2000.

The price of $1,000 a dose is probably a lowball estimate. Anesthesiologists, not just at Columbia, talk of a per-dose price in the $1,400 range. David Royston is the source for the background information on the drug's development and Bayer's current strategy, including the BSE-certified herds. (He is a regular speaker for aprotinin, and in close touch with the company.) The other fibrinolytics are well described in Mangano, *op. cit.*, and Karkouti, *op. cit.*

The Problem with Randomized Clinical Trials
Angell, *op. cit.*, pp. 99–111, for company manipulation of trials. For the 3.6 figure, see Justin Bekelman, "Scope and Impact of Financial Conflicts of Interest in Biomedical Research," *Journal of the American Medical Association* 289 (January 22,

2003): 454–486. For the fluoxetine example, see C. Barbu et al., "Fluoxetine Dose and Outcome in Antidepressant Drug Trials," *European Journal of Clinical Pharmacology* 58:6 (September 2002): 379–386. I learned a lot about RCTs and other statistical valuative methods from Sherry Glied, "Reviving the Dismal Science? Assessing the Value of Technological Improvements in Health Care," paper presented at the "Reassessing the Value Equation Conference," Boston, June 25, 2004. On RCTs in particular, see Samuel Shapiro, "Looking to the 21st Century: Have We Learned from Our Mistakes or Are We Doomed to Compound Them," *Pharmacoepidemiology and Drug Safety* 13:2 (February 2004): 257–265. For the meta-analysis of 8,500 cardiac patients, Philippe Gabriel Steg et al., "External Validity of Clinical Trials in Acute Myocardial Infarction," *Archives of Internal Medicine* 167:1 (January 8, 2007): 68–73. I also corresponded with one of the coauthors, Dr. Joel Gore, of the University of Massachusetts Medical Center. Sherwin Nuland's quotation is from an interview.

The Promise of Propensity Scoring

The description of propensity scoring and the challenge of observational databases rely primarily on Donald P. Rubin, "Estimating Causal Effects from Large Data Sets Using Propensity Scores," *Annals of Internal Medicine: Supplement on Statistical Methods* 127:8, pt. 2 (October 15, 1997): 757–763; and Ralph D'Agostino, "Propensity Score Methods for Bias Reduction in the Comparison of a Treatment to a Non-Randomized Control Group," *Statistics in Medicine*, 17:19 (October 15, 1998): 2265–2281. The "remarkably misleading" quote is from Rubin, p. 760. The Blackstone "it takes" is from Eugene H. Blackstone, "Comparing Apples and Oranges," *Journal of Thoracic and Cardiovascular Surgery* 123 (January 2002): 8–15, at 13. The 2002 Mangano paper is Dennis T. Mangano et al., "Aspirin and Mortality from Coronary Bypass Surgery," *New England Journal of Medicine* 347:17 (October 24, 2002): 1309–1317. Mangano's "shouldn't we" is from correspondence in the *New England Journal of Medicine* 354:18 (May 4, 2006): 1957.

The Problems of Propensity Scoring

See "Practice Guidelines for Perioperative Blood Transfusion and Adjuvant Therapies," *Anesthesiology* 105:1 (July 2006): 198–208. The aprotinin evidence is summarized at 205. The *New England Journal of Medicine* editorial "Randomized Trials or Observational Tribulations" appeared in vol. 342 (June 22, 2000): 1907–1909. The paper questioning quality of recent propensity studies is B. R. Shah, "Propensity Score Methods Gave Similar Results to Traditional Regression Modeling in Observational Studies: A Systematic Review," *Journal of Clinical Epidemiology* 58:6 (June 2005): 550–559. The Rubin message is from an email of August 17, 2006. Stan Young's "solely" is from an interview. German data are from the presentation "Outcomes Using Aprotinin Therapy" by Linda Shore-Lesserson at the September 2006 advisory committee hearing. The National Academy recommendations are from "Uniform Principles for Sharing Integral Data and Materials Expeditiously," *PNAS* 101:4 (March 16, 2004): 3721–3722. The "were offered limited" quote is from Dwaine Rieves, FDA Center for Drug Evaluation and Research, Cardiovascular and Renal Drugs Advisory Committee, Transcript of Morning Session, September 21, 2006, at p. 92 (hereafter "Transcript"). The "offered the FDA" is from the *New England Journal of Medicine* editorial "Research Replication," 355:21 (November 23, 2006): 2252–2253, at 2252. The related Mangano letter is at 2261–2262. For Karkouti study referenced in the note, see Karkouti, *op. cit.*

Soap Opera

For examples of Dr. Walker's methods, see, e.g, Andrew T. McAfee et al., "The Comparative Safety of Rosuvastatin: A Retrospective Matched Cohort Study in over 48,000 Initiators of

Stain Therapy," *Pharmacoepidemiology and Drug Safety* 15:6 (June 2006): 444–453; and Priscilla Velentgas et al., "Cardiovascular Risk of Selective Cyclooxygenase-2 Inhibitors and Other Non-aspirin Non-steroidal Anti-inflammatory Medications, *Pharmacoepidemiology and Drug Safety* 15:9 (September 2006): 641–652. I also had several email exchanges with Dr. Walker on his methods. Depending on the nature of the databases he is analyzing, he uses either propensity analyses or multiple regressions or both. In addition, specific adverse outcomes are always followed up with a full case review and are not included in study results unless they have been appropriately documented.

For the Bayer actions after the new study revelations, see the company press release "Bayer Appoints Independent Investigator to Review Trasylol Study Issues," October 13, 2006. The label changes are from a comparison of the 2000 label "Trasolyl® (aprotinin injection)," issued December 3, 2000, and the 2006 label of the same name issued December 15, 2006, both available from the FDA Web site. For a fairly complete history of Drazen's bumpy career at the *New England Journal of Medicine*, including the quotation "that medical journals" and the estimate of the *NEJM* profits, see Richard Smith, "Lapses at the *New England Journal of Medicine*," *Journal of the Royal Society of Medicine* 99 (August 2006): 1–3. The DeMets quote is from Transcript, Afternoon Session, 154–155.

Excerpts from September 2006 FDA Expert
Advisory Panel Hearing

The following exchanges are extracted from the dialog between Mangano and the advisory panel on the issue of data sharing (Transcript, Morning Session, 89–93):

John Flack (Panel): [To Mangano] I am impressed, though, and somewhat surprised, by your steadfast sort of conviction that this data is unassailable. We work with this kind of data all the time and I have never had that kind of conviction working with observational data, because there is too many problems that you can run into even with the best analytical techniques. . . .

[I]f you are this confident in the data and you want a body like this to render an opinion about how it should affect labeling in this, that and the other, then, when are you going to be prepared to make the data available to the scientists at least at the FDA? . . . [A]re you prepared now to basically let the FDA scientists analyze the data and go from there, because otherwise, I have serious reservations about what you are putting through here. . . .

Mangano: Okay. I offered the FDA the first week of February this database and I brought a CD and wanted to give it to them. I prepared CDs for the FDA to look at every single field in this database.

The FDA then wanted to combine this data with Bayer's data. Bayer also wanted my data. I purchased the computer with the entire database on it, brought it to the FDA and said, here, the only constraint is I want to be present when you are analyzing it and I want the data, because I am the custodian of the data, intellectual property, et cetera. You may not like that. I purchased the computer, I put the database on the computer, I gave it to the FDA.

F: That's not the way we do science.

M: What?

F: That's not the way we do science. Data is made available from the studies that the government funds and people are not necessarily there.

M: Well, isn't your question did I offer the FDA the database? I did. I would give it to them tomorrow.

F: Okay. There seems to be a difference of opinion, I guess—

M: I will show you the correspondence, I will show you the CDs prepared. I will bring the computer that I purchased and I will bring four people who came with me to the FDA at our expense to do that.

F: Well, I think the FDA is here and I think they can respond to this.

M: Okay, but, you know, that's—that's what it is.

William Hiatt (Chair): Any response?

Dwaine Rieves (FDA): We appreciate the comments there and that is correct. We were offered limited access to the data. There was this qualifying expectation that our examination be chaperoned or supervised, if you will.

Our statisticians did not feel comfortable with that limitation and, considering we have had fairly lengthy negotiations throughout the spring and early summer, our attorneys with other attorneys, that sort of thing, to try to obtain the data for, quote "somewhat of an independent," at least exploration of the mathematics. . . .

Our statisticians felt uncomfortable having a supervised access to that data in the sense that we would not have the ability to explore the data and at least verify the mathematics and the statistical aspects.

So, after a lot of negotiations during the spring, as well as during the summer, we decided that these were not going to be productive, meaning essentially that we were not going to have independent access or unsupervised access to the data set.

M: Well, in terms of the supervision, I would like to make a comment that all I required was that I be physically present within the FDA when you were analyzing the data. There is—I am sorry—there are patient confidentialities here that are important, that I respect.

Flack: This data, number one, is large. Two, it should be de-identified where nobody can link that data to a patient and, three, I don't understand, what do you think being present in the building is going to accomplish in regards to safeguarding the integrity of the science or confidentiality. That escapes me.

M: You have an opinion and it has obviously been weighted to some degree before this meeting.

F: No, I do science all the time.

M: All I can say is that I am happy to share this data.

Hiatt: Perhaps we won't debate that further maybe.

[Later, under questioning from another committee member, Mangano seemed to change his position somewhat. (Transcript, Morning Session, 114–115.)]

M: . . . We offered to work with the FDA and it didn't happen. We will offer to work with them again. But we— you know, this is a new paradigm in terms of independent data being shared and contrasted. . . . So, the question is, one of the major questions that came up is if you are going to do a meta-analysis of everything and put everything into a pot, what is the design of that study, what are your endpoints, what are your questions, because you could pull out anything you want. . . .

    You could take this data and pull out anything you want out of it. You could say the drug is safe and don't ever worry about it again, but if the FDA is going to perform a series of analyses, we believe it important to get the design for those analyses presented to us in written form, so we know what the prospective question is, because don't forget, the FDA is under some pressure right here, which is that they have a drug that is marketed 13 years.

[The transcript shows no reaction from committee members or staff to Mangano's offer, if that's what it was, which is hardly surprising. Months of negotiation had already taken place over release of the data, and Mangano's suggestion, along with its implication of bad faith at the FDA, would seem to open the door to yet more months of fruitless negotiation over the types of analyses that would be acceptable.]

Chapter 8: THE FUTURE OF HEART SURGERY

Trends in use of cardiac and cardiovascular procedures from 1993 to 2003 were calculated by me from the Center for Disease Control, "National Hospitals Discharge Survey for 2003," released in 2005. Population adjustments were calculated from U.S. Census data. The "one million" figure for stent placements in 2006 is from the *New York Times*, December 6, 2006. Medicare rate data were supplied by Ellen B. Griffith of the Federal Centers for Medicare and Medicaid Services. The Web posting on reduced opportunities for surgeons was dated June 8, 2005. The poster was Atiq Rehman, of Columbus, Mississippi. CTSNet is the Web site for the Society of Cardiovascular and Thoracic Surgeons. My appreciation to Doris Stoll of the American Council on Graduate Medical Education and to Jennifer Quill, program manager at Columbia-Presbyterian, for their assistance in collecting the resident data. On drug-eluting stents, "more than 80 percent of all placements" is in Mark Jewell, "Boston Scientific's Stent Sales Fall," AP, January 10, 2007. For a careful summary of the business background of DES, see "Drug-Eluting Stents: A Paradigm Shift in the Medical Device Industry," *Stanford Graduate School of Business, Case OIT-50*, February 13, 2006.

The criticisms of the DES first erupted at the World Congress of Cardiology held in Barcelona in September 2006. A Web-based resource, theheart.org, a service of WebMD, provided daily dispatches: "Studies Linking Drug-Eluting Stents to Increased Mortality/MI Spark Impassioned Pleas for Reason and Calls for Calm," September 3, 2006. Dr. Salim Yusuf, of McMaster University in Toronto, a much-published cardiologist and researcher, is the "epidemic" speaker; see also "Yusuf, Serruys Square Off over DES in Chronic Stable Angina," September 5, 2006. Some worries were surfacing well before the conference, however: "Palpable Chill Cools DES Hype, but Hopes are High for Next-Generation Devices," May 19, 2006. Data on DES usage trends are from a Leon presentation, "The Current State of Drug-Eluting Stents," American College of Cardiology Scientific Session, New Orleans, March, 2007. For the December FDA recommendation, see "FDA Advisory Panel on the Safety and Efficacy of Drug Eluting Stents: Summary of Findings and Recommendations," see www.fda.gov/cdrh/panel/summary/circ-120706.html. The full report is available at www.theheart.org. For a careful review of the advisory committee's proceedings, see Miriam Schuchman, "Debating the Risks of Drug-Eluting Stents," *New England Journal of Medicine* 356:4 (January 25, 2007): 325–327. For "modest effect," see Mark Jewell, *op. cit.*

The history of PVT is based on my interview with Stan Rabinovich and company materials. The first-round trial results were presented at the TCT conference by Leon, but have not yet been published at this writing.

Chapter 9: MONEY

The estimates of private cardiac surgeons' earnings are from a Web forum sponsored by the Stanford Medical School. On specialty hospitals in general, see the collection of articles in *Health Affairs* January–February 2006, esp. Stuart Guterman, "Specialty Hospitals: A Problem or a Symptom," 95–105; and Jeffrey Stensland et al., "Do Physician-Owned Hospitals Increase Utilization," 119–129. The criticism of Columbia medical faculty salaries was in the *New York Sun*, May 26, 2005. The Shaw quote is in George Khusuf et al., "Understanding, Assessing, and Managing Conflicts of Interest, in Lawrence B. McCullough et al., eds., *Surgical Ethics* (New York: Oxford University Press), pp. 343–366, at 344. For the ethical framework described in the note, see *ibid.*, pp. 350–355, and for self-referral rate in owned radiology services, *ibid.*, p. 351. The spinal fusion business model is from "The Spine As Profit Center," *New York Times*, December 30, 2006. For thoughtful analyses of the interaction between academic medical centers and industry, see Annetine Gelijns et al., "Evidence, Politics, and Technological Change," *Health Affairs* 24:1 (January-February 2005): 29–40; and Annetine Gelijns et al., "The Dynamics of Technological Change in Medicine," *Health Affairs* (Summer 1994), 28–46. Columbia patent data through 1995 is from David C. Mowery, "The Changing Role of Universities in the 21st-Century U.S. R&D System," in David C. Mowery et al., eds., *Paths of Innovation: Technological Change in 20th-Century America* (New York: Cambridge University Press), pp. 253–271, at 266. Update through 2005 is from Columbia University Science and Technology Ventures, *Annual Report 2005*.

Chapter 10: POLICY

The 30 percent figure within twenty years is on the high side of current estimates, but most official estimates have consistently underestimated the actual growth rate. The 30 percent is derived from the projections in Victor R. Fuchs, "Provide, Provide: The Economics of Aging," NBER Working Paper No. 6642, July 1998. If this estimate is in fact too high, then the problems of accommodating health care's growth will be even simpler than described here. The expedited 2002 approval process for stents is from 'Drug-Eluting Stents: A Paradigm Shift in the Medical Device Industry, *Stanford Graduate School of Business, Case*

OIT-50, February 13, 2006, p. 18. For the Ford-Schultz comments, see William Clay Ford, "Speech Before the U.S. Chamber of Commerce," November 10, 2004, and "Health Care Takes Its Toll on Starbucks," MSNBC, September 14, 2005. The sectoral economic shifts are well laid out in Robert William Fogel, *The Escape from Hunger and Premature Death, 1700–2100: Europe, America, and the Third World* (New York: Cambridge University Press, 2004), an important book. See also, "Factory Jobs Are Becoming Scarce; It's Nothing to Worry About," *The Economist*, September 29, 2005. For the research data on American doctors and care standards, see the findings of Allison B. Rosen, M.D., et al., "Physicians' Views of Interventions to Reduce Medical Errors: Does Evidence of Effectiveness Matter?" *Academic Medicine* 80 (February 2005): 189–192; Charles P. Friedman et al., "Do Physicians Know When Their Diagnoses Are Correct?" *Journal of General Internal Medicine* 20 (April 2005): 334–339; Anne-Marie J. Audet, M.D., et al., "Findings from the Commonwealth Fund National Survey of Physicians and the Quality of Care," The Commonwealth Fund, May 2005; Christopher L. Roy et al., "Patient Safety Concerns Arising from Test Results That Return After Hospital Discharge," *Improving Patient Care* 143:2 (July 19, 2005): 121–128; Anne-Marie Audet et al., "Measure, Learn, and Improve: Physicians' Involvement in Quality Improvement," *Health Affairs*, May–June 2005: 843–853; Commonwealth Fund, "Issue of the Month: Chronic Disease Management in Medicare," June 2005; Cathy Schoen et al., "U.S. Health System Performance: A National Scorecard," *Health Affairs* (Web exclusive, September 20, 2006), W457–475; Cathy Schoen et al., "On the Front Lines of Care: Primary Care Doctors' Office Systems: Experiences and Views in Seven Countries," *Health Affairs* (Web exclusive, November 2, 2006), W555–571; Jonathan S. Skinner et al., "Is Technological Change in Medicine Always Worth It? The Case of Acute Myocardial Infarction," *Health Affairs* (Web exclusive, February 7, 2006), W34–27. The data on federal research spending is from *U.S.*

Budget, 2007: Analytical Perspectives, p. 49, Table 5-1; cumulative health research spending is from Elias Zerhouni, "Testimony Before the Senate Subcommittee on Labor—HHS—Education Appropriations," May 19, 2006. (I converted Zerhouni's per capita numbers.) American and European stent usage is from "Drug-Eluting Stents," Stanford Graduate School of Business, *op. cit,* p. 8, and for the Guidant executive quote (Guido Neels, COO in 2004), p. 4. For slower cutbacks in U.S., see Mark Jewell, "Boston Scientific's Stent Sales Fall," AP, January 10, 2007. Both theheart.org and TCT Web sites have multiple CME programs on stents. Leon's pullback recommendation is from his "The Current State of Drug-Eluting Stents," American College of Cardiology Scientific Session, New Orleans, March, 2007. The Cutler quote is from David M. Cutler, "Making Sense of Medical Technology," *Health Affairs* (Web exclusive, February 7, 2006), W48–50, at W48 . The Leonhardt quote is from David Leonhardt, "What Money Doesn't Buy in Health Care," *New York Times*, December 13, 2006.

Appendix I: HOW THE HEART WORKS

For a compact introductory text, see, for example, David E. Newby and Neil R. Grubb, *Cardiology* (Edinburgh, U.K.: Elsevier, 2005).

Appendix II: THE NEW YORK STATE CARDIAC HOSPITAL RATING SYSTEM

The NYS and U.S. comparative data are from a presentation delivered by Ed Hannan at Columbia-Presbyterian on September 21, 2006. I calculated the comparison table from the State Department of Health reports, "Adult Cardiac Surgery in New York State," for the ten years covered. My appreciation to Larry Beilis for checking my table.

INDEX

Page numbers in *italics* refer to illustrations.

ABOUT THE AUTHOR

CHARLES R. MORRIS HAS WRITTEN TEN BOOKS, including *The Cost of Good Intentions*, one of the *New York Times*'s Ten Best Books of 1980; *The Coming Global Boom*, a *New York Times* Notable Book of 1990; *Computer Wars* (with Charles H. Ferguson) one of *Business Week*'s Best Books of 1993; and *The Tycoons*, a *Barron's* Best Book of 2005. He is a lawyer and has also been a banker and investment banker. Mr. Morris's articles and reviews have appeared in the *Atlantic Monthly*, the *New York Times Magazine*, the *Harvard Business Review*, the *New York Times*, the *Wall Street Journal*, and many other publications. He is a member of the Council on Foreign Relations and lives in New York City.